# So you have Diabetes!

# So you have
# Diabetes!

## Larry A. Distiller

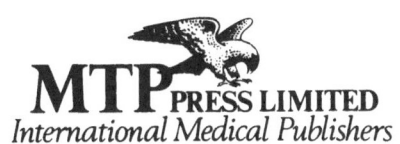
MTP PRESS LIMITED
*International Medical Publishers*

Published by
MTP Press Limited
Falcon House
Lancaster, England

Copyright © 1980 L. A. Distiller
Softcover reprint of the hardcover 1st edition 1980

First published 1980

**British Library Cataloguing in Publication Data**

Distiller, Larry A.
  So you have diabetes!
  1.  Diabetes
  I.  Title
    616.4'62     RC660

ISBN-13: 978-94-011-6240-1    e-ISBN-13: 978-94-011-6238-8
DOI: 10.1007/978-94-011-6238-8

# Contents

# A note from the author

Many books written for the diabetic start with a statement such as 'a diabetic can lead a perfectly normal life', and then go on to give a long list of do's and do not's, must's and must not's, can's and cannot's, so that at the end of it the diabetic is left with the conclusion that a perfectly normal life, for a diabetic, consists of a regimented, jailed and restricted lifestyle with all the fun, enjoyment and spontaneity removed. In fact, a diabetic *can* lead a perfectly normal life with only minimal important alterations in lifestyle. In order to do this, the single most important factor is a complete understanding of diabetes. Several years of dealing with diabetics from all walks of life have made me realize that the majority of diabetic patients know far too little about their disease. This results in their having to restrict their lives and activities because they do not understand how to cope with their bodies' response to even minor deviations in day-to-day living. This has prompted me to write this short book, attempting to explain the necessary principles and guidelines in a language that can be understood by any intelligent adult without scientific or medical training. No attempt has been made to provide absolute or detailed academic accuracy, and since this book deals with principles only, I have purposefully excluded long lists of recommended diets and food exchange.

LARRY A. DISTILLER

# Acknowledgements

Many people were instrumental in making this book a reality. In the first instance, my grateful thanks go to my wife Brenda and our three children for sacrificing our time together so that this book could become a reality. Dr Barry Joffe, Professor Harry Seftel, and Dr Everard Polakow all read the manuscript, supplying useful advice and constructive criticism. I thank them for their time. I must express my deep appreciation to my secretary, Miss Kathy Rosenberg, for her dedication and efficiency in the typing and retyping of this manuscript. My appreciation also goes to the many diabetic patients who, over the years, have made me realize the importance of self-education in overall diabetic control. Many of my patients were aware of the conception of this book and their constant encouragement was a persistent stimulus to me.

# Introduction

Diabetes is one of the oldest diseases known to mankind. It was first mentioned in the Ebers Payrus (Egypt 1500 BC) and 'honey urine' was noted by Sushrutha in India in 400 BC. By the first century of the Christian era the disease was well known, both in Roman writings and in Chinese and Japanese writings. The word 'diabetes' was first coined by the Greeks. It means a passing-through of water. They described it as a 'melting of flesh into water', meaning urine. Then in 1674 Doctor Willis discovered by heating, tasting and evaporating urine that a sweet sticky substance was in it, which, of course, was sugar. But sugar was not known in England in those days and honey was the only real sweet tasting substance. The Latin word 'mel' which means honey was used and the disease came to be known as diabetes mellitus – that is, the passing of honeyed urine. This is still the full name of the disease.

Over the next few centuries, treatment by means of dieting was started but nothing important was discovered to solve the problem of diabetes. In 1889 two Germans, experimenting on the effect of removing the pancreas gland on the digestion of dogs, discovered that the animals developed diabetes. The dogs became thirsty, the bottoms of their cages were sticky with sugar and they died in a coma. Thus, it was realized that removal of the pancreas in some way caused diabetes but the exact relationship was not understood until the discovery of insulin by Banting and Best.

Banting was a 28-year-old surgeon who after being seriously wounded in the World War of 1914–1918, returned to

Canada to practice and teach surgery. One night, while reading and preparing a lecture on the pancreas and diabetes, he developed an idea. After some difficulties with the authorities, he was finally given a laboratory, permission to operate on dogs, and an assistant to do the work of chemical analysis; this was Charles Best, a final year medical student of 21 years. And so they came to work together, these two men whose research was to lead to combined and shared success. But their path to success was not easy. The early experiments went wrong, money ran short, and they sold personal belongings to buy materials that they needed. After several months of exhaustive work they managed to produce an extract from the pancreas which brought down the raised blood sugar in a diabetic dog. After another few months, this extract was shown to have the same effect on people with diabetes. After scores of other experiments it was discovered how to extract insulin from the pancreas of cattle killed for food, and this remains the major source of insulin available for use.

The breakthrough engineered by Banting and Best completely altered the outlook for persons with diabetes. Since then world-wide interest in diabetes has been sustained. and many advances have been made in the treatment of diabetes and its complications. This is as it should be, since diabetes is an extremely common and unfortunately irreversible disease. On the basis of many surveys, it is estimated that at least one person in 50 in the Western World has diabetes. This amounts to more than 4 000 000 persons in the United States of America alone. It is believed that in almost half of these persons the condition is not recognized for various reasons such as individual neglect, the mildness or even absence of symptoms, and inadequate medical care. It is probably reasonable to assess further that 25% of the population, or roughly 50 000 000 people in the United States of America, either have diabetes, will develop diabetes, or have a diabetic relative. The disease therefore poses a problem for a large number of people, either directly or indirectly.

# Chapter One

## *What is diabetes?*

The human body derives its energy from the food which it eats. Basically, there are three general food stuffs: carbohydrates, proteins and fats.

In the intestinal tract starches and sugars (carbohydrates) are broken down and converted to a simple sugar – glucose. Proteins are broken down to their structural elements – amino acids. Fats are split into fatty acids. In the cells of the body, glucose, amino acids and fatty acids are again broken down to carbon dioxide, water, nitrogen and minerals, and by this process energy is released. We use this released energy for heating our bodies, for building other complex chemical structures, for muscle action, and in fact for all the necessary functions of life. It is mainly the glucose and the fatty acids which we use for energy; the protein breakdown products, known as amino acids, are used as 'building blocks' (Figure 1). Only in starvation and uncontrolled diabetes are proteins broken down for energy. The whole range of chemical reactions is carefully co-ordinated to provide a smoothly functioning body and this is an enormously complex process.

Therefore, glucose is the basis of all carbohydrates and is found in 'starchy' foods, such as wheat, potatoes, and rice. Generally, these foods, which have a high carbohydrate content, are the cheap and filling foods, and are therefore the staple food of most populations. Glucose is also present to some extent in fruit, together with another slightly different sugar known as fructose. However, we find glucose in its most concentrated form (sucrose) in refined sugar. This is the sort of

1

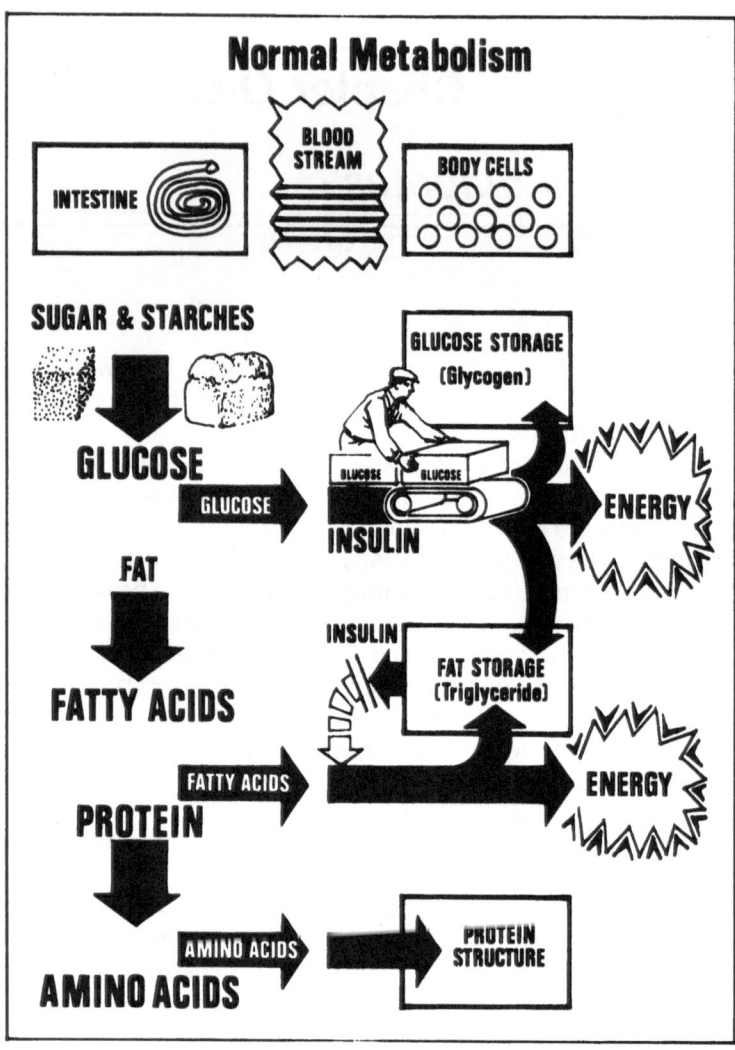

**Figure 1**

sugar found in candies, cakes and sweetened carbonated drinks.

A certain basic amount of glucose is necessary in the diet, but ideally this should be in the form of natural sugars (e.g. starch, fruit) and not in the form of refined sugars (sucrose).

Once glucose enters the bloodstream, the body burns up as much as it needs for immediate energy. Any excessive amounts of glucose are then stored as triglyceride (body fat) both in the liver and the fat stores of the body or as glycogen in the liver. This process of glucose usage and storage is very complicated, and one of the most important factors in this process is the hormone, insulin. Insulin is essential for the breakdown of glucose to energy and for the storage of fat and glycogen (see Figure 1). Insulin also prevents excessive fat (triglyceride) breakdown so that it promotes the storage of energy.

If one does not eat for a period of time, fat and protein stores are broken down to release the stored energy. Insulin prevents this process from taking place, while other hormones, such as adrenaline and growth hormone, promote it. Where fat is broken down in large amounts for energy, one of the by-products formed is acetone (see Figure 2).

Insulin is normally secreted by the pancreas in response to rising blood glucose levels or in response to food intake in general, so that insulin levels are highest when one has just eaten and lowest when fasting. The relationship of insulin to other hormones tends to ensure that the normal level of glucose in the blood remains remarkably constant in most individuals, and whether one fasts for a long period or eats a large meal, fluctuation of glucose in the blood is minimal. The amount of glucose in the blood can be measured in the laboratory and the level is usually expressed as milligrams of glucose in 100 millilitres of blood (mg%). Recently, there has been a trend to express the blood glucose level in a new way, as SI units, or millimoles per litre. Normally, after not eating for at least 5 hours, the blood glucose level varies between 60 and 110 mg% (3.4 to 6.2 mmol/l). This is known as a fasting blood

3

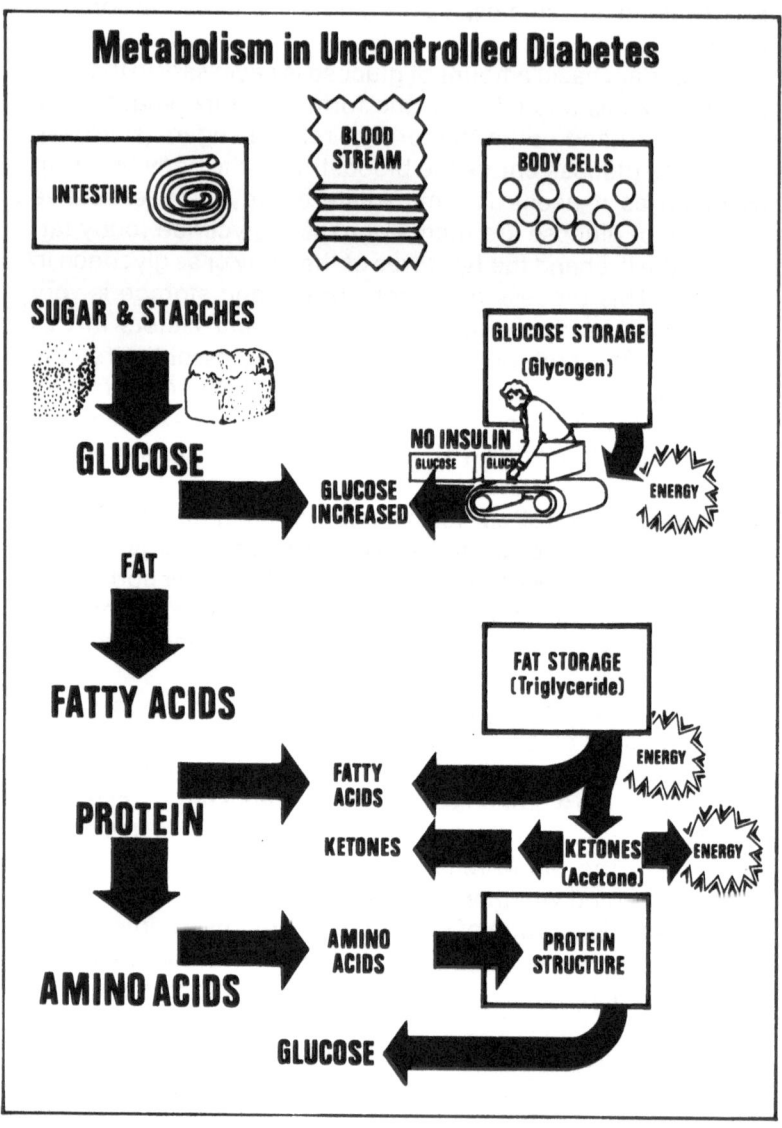

**Figure 2**

sugar. Under normal circumstances, the glucose in the blood never rises above 160 mg% (9 mmol/l) even after eating.

The circulating pool of glucose in the blood is maintained as an immediate source of energy for minute-by-minute living, whereas that stored as fat or glycogen acts as a reserve of fuel. If the quantity of insulin produced is too little to allow for glucose to be used, or to be stored, glucose accumulates in the blood, especially after meals. Therefore, the hall-mark of diabetes, which is due to an insulin deficiency, is a rapid increase in the level of glucose in the blood to more than normal amounts after meals. If there is a large deficiency in the amount of insulin needed, the reserves of fuel in the liver and fat tissue are broken down unrestrainedly, releasing more glucose into the bloodstream. This results in a wasteful situation where the body is unable to store energy and even breaks down protein to produce excess glucose (Figure 2). The severity of the insulin deficiency determines the severity of the diabetes. If there is only a slight deficiency, the disturbance is relatively mild and the only manifestation may be a high blood glucose content after consumption of sugar. However, if the insulin deficiency is severe, the blood glucose will not only be high after meals but will be high between meals. If the insulin deficiency is extremely severe, the blood will become choked with fatty acids and their breakdown products – ketones.

The kidney, which is a large self-adjusting filter, does not normally allow any precious energy-giving glucose to be lost, and therefore no sugar is excreted in the urine. However, if the blood glucose rises too high, usually above 180 mg% (10 mmol/l), the kidneys are no longer able to hold the sugar back and it 'spills over' into the urine. This never happens in the normal individual (without diabetes) unless the kidney is faulty and allows glucose to overflow into the urine at blood sugar levels lower than 180 mg%; this occurs in about 5% of the normal population, who are said to have 'glycosuria without diabetes'. (Glycosuria simply means sugar in the urine.)

Diabetes can be divided roughly into two groups:

(1) *Juvenile onset diabetes* This occurs in young people, usually under the age of 30 years, who develop diabetes because the pancreas is unable to produce enough insulin and the insulin deficiency is usually marked. Therefore, these diabetics always require insulin as treatment.

(2) *Maturity onset diabetes* This occurs in people who develop diabetes over the age of 40 years, and most of them are overweight. These patients can frequently be treated without insulin.

Because of the deficiency of insulin in diabetes, the glucose that is eaten cannot be used as energy, nor can it be stored. Therefore the glucose level in the blood increases. This can be compared to a 'go-slow' or strike by workers in a factory. The raw material (glucose) enters the factory but is not incorporated into the end product because of the failure of the workers (insulin). The raw material therefore just mounts up on the factory floor until it overflows from the building. This happens in diabetes, and as the blood sugar rises progressively it finally exceeds the kidney threshhold; that is, it spills over into the urine. In order to excrete the sugar, the urine has to be diluted (or else one would urinate syrup – a slow, inconvenient and somewhat messy alternative!). More water is therefore excreted by the kidney. This results in a large increase in urine volume so that there develops a frequent passing of large volumes of urine, during the day and the night. Passing so much urine can cause a fairly rapid degree of dehydration which then results in a dry mouth and unquenchable thirst, symptoms well known to any diabetic (Figure 3).

Prolonged high blood sugar levels are associated with insufficient glucose being used for energy production and therefore the diabetic feels tired and weak. At the same time there is a breakdown of fat and protein (muscle) in the body in an attempt to find other sources of energy. This results in weight loss and further weakness. Finally, if the insulin deficiency is severe enough there is an acute energy shortage, ketone levels begin to rise in the blood and this will show in the urine. Ketones, a by-product of emergency energy production

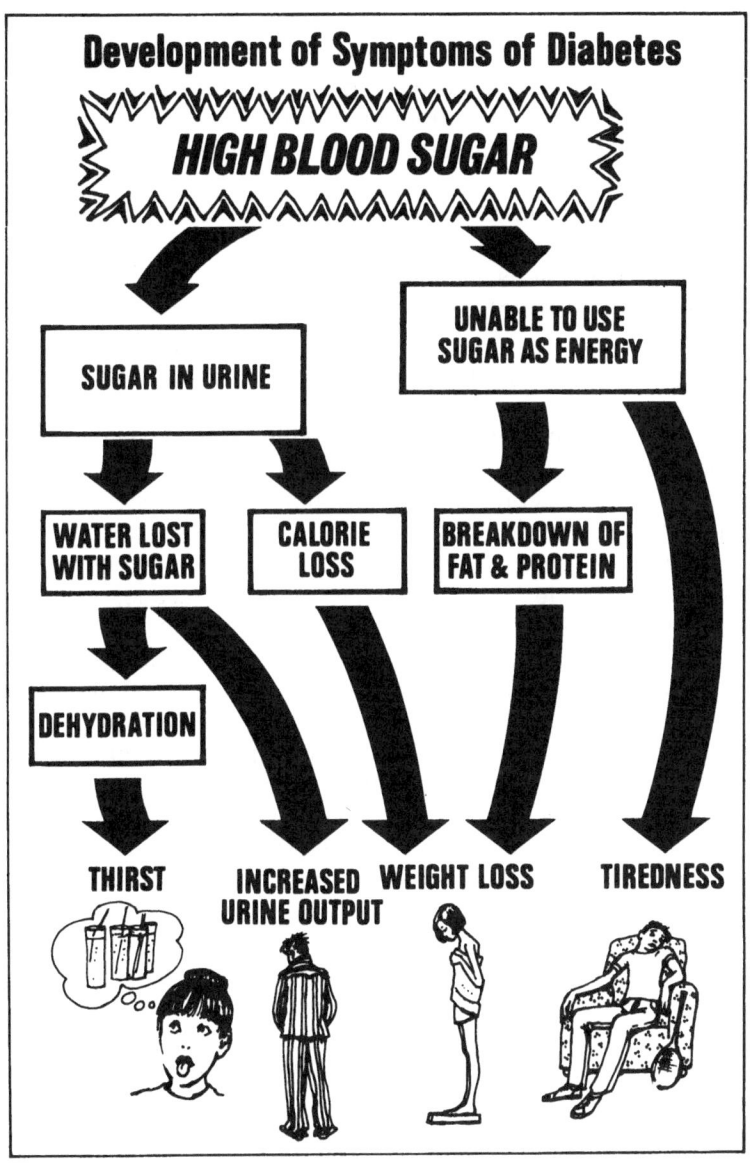

**Figure 3**

7

from fat, are acids and will make the blood too acidic. This can cause nausea, vomiting, abdominal upsets, shortness of breath and confusion. Furthermore, since the brain *must* have glucose for normal functioning, if the diabetic state gets bad enough, the brain may suffer from lack of energy and coma may ensue.

Alterations in blood sugar, such as are found in the uncontrolled diabetic state, cause a certain swelling and contracting of the lens of the eye which can result in various degrees of blurring of vision. This can also happen to the balance apparatus in the inner ear, so that at times the uncontrolled diabetic may suffer from intermittent dizziness and loss of balance.

The majority of diabetics fit into the maturity onset group, and most of these people are overweight. In many of these diabetics there is only a *relative* deficiency of insulin, which is still produced in normal amounts by the pancreas. Basically, an increase in fat tissue is associated with an increased resistance to the action of insulin on the fat tissue, liver and muscle. Therefore fat people need much more insulin than normal to use, burn up or store available glucose. If the pancreas is normal, it can cope with the increased demands and this is what happens with most obese, non-diabetic individuals. On the other hand, if there is an inherent problem in the pancreas so that it cannot cope with the increased demands placed upon it, the insulin production is insufficient and diabetes ensues. This is usually a milder form of diabetes, found in older people. Again, the analogy of the factory can be used. The situation in the obese maturity onset diabetic can be likened to a factory which is operating on skeleton staff only. As long as the raw material entering the factory is not excessive, the workers can cope with the work load. However, because of an excessive supply of raw material (glucose) the workers (insulin) are overworked. The raw material will again mount up on the factory floor until it overflows from the building, but this is due to a slightly different sequence of events from that depicted (above) in the juvenile diabetic.

Diabetes may occur in many degrees, and depending on

the severity, diabetes may be graded as chemical, latent or overt. Initially, the fasting (resting) blood sugar may be normal, and diabetes may only be shown by loading the patient with glucose (a glucose tolerance test), which may show that the body cannot produce enough insulin in response to the glucose load and the blood sugar level rises excessively and transiently. This is the mildest form of diabetes and is known as *chemical diabetes*. Then there is the sort of diabetes in which the blood sugar increases at the time of severe stress such as illness or pregnancy or when a person is given cortisone medication. This is called *latent diabetes* which suggests that the person is likely to develop true diabetes at a later stage in his life. Finally, there is *overt diabetes* when both the fasting blood sugar and the blood sugar after glucose ingestion is abnormally elevated. This is true diabetes which may be mild enough not to be recognized or may reveal itself through symptoms of thirst, frequency of urination, weakness, blurring of vision and weight loss. If it is very severe, ketones may be produced in large amounts causing nausea, loss of appetite, stomach pains and shortness of breath and the patient may even lose consciousness; this is called diabetic ketoacidosis.

There are many causes of diabetes. The majority of cases are spontaneous (also known as hereditary, idiopathic, primary or essential diabetes) and some ideas on the development of this sort of diabetes are considered in the next chapter. Occasionally, diabetes may be due to actual damage to the pancreas, induced by alcohol, trauma or surgery, and even more rarely it could be due to overproduction or administration of hormones antagonistic to insulin, such as cortisone, growth hormone or adrenalin.

Recently, another hormone produced by the pancreas and called glucagon has been incriminated in the overall picture of diabetes. The great majority of diabetics not only have decreased insulin levels but also increased glucagon produced by the pancreas. It is not definitely known what stimilates glucagon overproduction, but in almost every function glucagon acts against insulin. Therefore, in diabetes there is both an insulin deficiency and a glucagon excess. This is a

9

relatively new discovery and is receiving much attention, thought and research in current diabetic medical literature. It does not alter the basic principles of treating and managing diabetes at this stage, because when insulin is given to a diabetic, there is a fall in glucagon levels.

It is very important to realize that diabetes is by no means a disorder of glucose alone. Although, as already outlined, the inability to use and store glucose is the major problem, there are several other associated problems. In particular, because of the overall disturbance, there is a tendency towards high blood levels of fats. In particular, the fat known as triglyceride is often elevated, and the cholesterol level may also be raised. Both these fats are thought to play an important role in causing atheroma – fatty plaques on the walls of many arteries. As the fatty plaques increase they eventually cause the arteries to narrow and harden. They also cause roughening of the walls of the arteries which promotes blood clotting (thrombosis) in the affected vessels. The overall result is that the blood flow through these arteries is impeded and this can result in poor circulation to the legs. coronary thrombosis and strokes. as well as high blood pressure. Therefore, if you have diabetes you must consider the blood fats as well as the blood sugar in your overall management.

Summary

(1) Glucose is the most important food for energy.

(2) Glucose is stored as glycogen and body fat (triglycerides).

(3) Insulin is required for the utilization and storage of glucose.

(4) Diabetes is due to a deficiency of insulin, which causes high levels of glucose in the blood.

(5) In young diabetics, the insulin deficiency is usually severe, and insulin is usually required for treatment. In older

diabetics, the insulin deficiency is often milder, and treatment may take the form of diet with or without tablets.

(6) When the amount of glucose in the blood increases beyond a certain level, the glucose is passed in the urine and this causes most of the symptoms of diabetes.

(7) Diabetes has many causes, but the majority are spontaneous.

(8) In diabetes, the blood fats (cholesterol and triglycerides) are raised. This can damage the arteries. Therefore, blood fat levels must be considered in the overall management of diabetes.

# Chapter Two

## *The inheritance of diabetes*

Two factors are involved in the development of diabetes. These are heredity and the environment. We all accept that heredity plays a part in the onset of diabetes and it is doubtful whether environmental factors have ever caused diabetes in the absence of this inherited component. In most diabetics, heredity plays the major role. The familial tendency of diabetes was first noted in India as long ago as the seventh century. The exact pattern of the inheritance of diabetes has never been fully understood, because the pattern of inheritance is extremely complex. It was only in 1929 that it was noted that diabetes was very commonly found affecting both in a set of identical twins. If one identical twin has maturity onset diabetes, there is a greater than 60% chance that the other twin will develop maturity onset diabetes. Furthermore, a high percentage of children born to two diabetic parents will develop diabetes by 40 years of age.

Although the pattern of inheritance still remains a mystery, it appears in general as though juvenile onset diabetes and maturity onset diabetes have different types of inheritance, and that juvenile onset diabetes itself may have at least two or three quite distinct different inheritance patterns. Certainly, the inheritance factor in maturity onset diabetes is far stronger than in juvenile onset diabetes. If one parent has maturity onset diabetes, the chance of one of their children developing diabetes may be as high as 40%. On the other hand, the child of one juvenile onset diabetic parent has only a 1% chance of being a juvenile onset diabetic. If one parent and one child has juvenile onset diabetes, the chance of a second child being diabetic increases up to 15%. From time to time one comes across families where the inherited component in diabetes appears to be very strong. In one family the youngest daughter, aged 16 years, became diabetic, followed 6 months later by her elder sister, 1 year later by a third child, a brother and then weeks later by the mother. They had a large piece of paper tacked behind the bathroom door with an intricate table of their individual urine glucose tests. Mornings and evenings, chaos reined with all of them vying with each other for a place in the line for urine testing. They made quite a family game out of it and the father, the only non-diabetic member of the family, felt quite out of things. Fortunately, this is rather a rare situation, and two insulin-requiring diabetics in one family are not common. One man, aged 32 years, had recently married. He had become diabetic while serving in Viet-Nam and had developed a particularly bitter outlook. He requested sterilization by vasectomy because he did not want to 'pass on the gene' and despite prolonged discussions during which the chances of inheritance were explained to him, and even though his wife desperately wanted a child, he was adamant in his conviction. He finally managed to find a doctor to perform the vasectomy. This was, of course, a totally unrealistic attitude on behalf of the patient.

It must be accepted that a large number of people who inherit the tendency to develop diabetes never become diabetic. Thus, once one has inherited the diabetic tendency, a second environmental factor is necessary to cause diabetes to develop. It is difficult to know exactly what the inherited factor is which finally causes the diabetes. Available information suggests that it may be a basic defect in the production or release of insulin. In other cases it may be a problem in the body's immunity so that at a certain time of life the body stops recognizing the Islets of Langerhans (the insulin-producing cells in the pancreas) as belonging to itself, thinks of it as a foreign tissue, and therefore rejects and destroys the insulin-producing cells. Despite inheriting this tendency, the patient may never develop overt diabetes; this will depend on several environmental factors, some known, some suspected and some still unknown. The important environmental factors that we know precipitate diabetes in a susceptible individual are:

(1) *Pancreatic damage* This can be from alcohol or iron deposited in the pancreas. These substances can damage the pancreas and if the basic diabetic tendency is present, precipitate diabetes. Damage to the pancreas by accidents, blows to the abdomen, etc. is not thought to play a major part in precipitating diabetes.

(2) *Obesity* It has been said that heredity loads the gun but obesity and other stresses pull the trigger. It has been felt, particularly in maturity onset diabetes, that obesity is the most common precipitating cause and patients above 50 years of age seldom acquire overt diabetes if their weight remains a little below normal. In contrast, the greater the obesity the higher the incidence of diabetes.

(3) *Emotional factors* Many of the problems related to the onset of diabetes have to do with mental trauma, shock or emotional crises and upsets. However, the whole act of living in modern times is stressful, so that the exact role of stress in precipitating diabetes is difficult to evaluate. Still, it is likely that intense stress, particularly if prolonged, can finally tip the scale in favour of diabetes causing it to develop in a person predisposed to the condition. One little girl was apparently a healthy child until her parents were involved in a motor vehicle accident severely injuring both of them. While they were in hospital, she was sent to stay with a relative of whom she was not particularly fond. One week later this child developed severe sudden diabetes, necessitating hospital admission and insulin. Although her parents have subsequently recovered completely, the diabetes, of course, has remained. Many diabetics will date the onset of their diabetes to a sudden emotional or a physical shock, and blame their illness on the incident or person who caused the upset. In such an instance, it is worth remembering that the diabetic tendency was there,

lurking just beneath, and it would have manifested itself sooner or later anyway.

(4) *Virus infections* Recently the possibility of a mild virus infection of the pancreas being responsible for the onset of diabetes in genetically predisposed persons has been suggested. At present the evidence points towards this as a possibility, and it may occur far more frequently than previously thought, particularly in juvenile onset diabetes. Much work is now being conducted to determine the exact role of viral infections and to isolate the exact virus which is responsible.

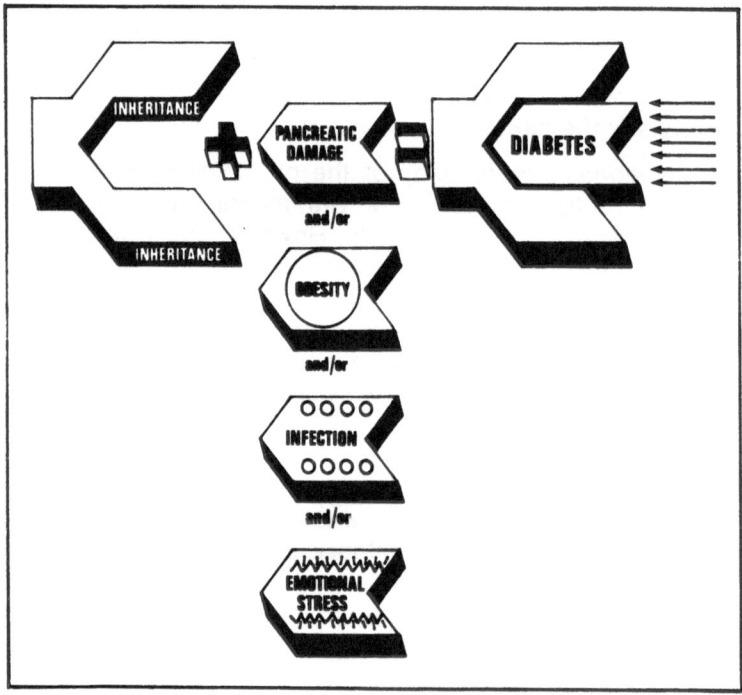

**Figure 4**

(5) *Other infections* It has been known for a long time that the stress of any infection, particularly if severe, may precipitate overt diabetes. Many other types of acute physical stress have been known to do this, such as strokes, myocardial infarction (cardiac thrombosis) or pregnancy (see Chapter 8).

In summary, it can be said that heredity is by far the most important factor in the development of diabetes mellitus, although the exact type of inheritance cannot be defined as yet. Once the genetic tendency is present, other environmental factors such as obesity, infection or intense emotional stress are needed to make the diabetes overt (see Figure 4).

# Chapter Three

## *Diet and diabetes*

The cornerstone of treatment in diabetes is undoubtedly diet, irrespective of the severity of the diabetes or the age of onset. However, the principles of diet vary between the diabetic on insulin and the diabetic controlled on diet alone or with tablets. For this reason, the two groups will be dealt with separately. General considerations pertaining to all diabetics, are discussed at the end of the chapter. The purpose of this section is purely to discuss the principles of diet without giving specific dietary advice. Individual diets should be prescribed by a doctor, and where possible this should be handled in conjunction with a trained dietician. If this is not possible, many books outlining specific calorie intakes and diets are readily available. Some suggested diets are included, for completeness, in the appendices at the end of this book.

Insulin-requiring diabetics

As outlined in Chapter 1, this sort of diabetic has one basic problem – a deficiency of insulin. The deficiency has been corrected by giving insulin. If the patient is of normal weight there is therefore no need to restrict calories. The great majority of people keep their weight remarkably stable over the months and years by inherently controlling food intake, and there is no reason why, if diabetes develops, this basic instinct should be lost. In fact, the total calories and the proportions of starch, fat and protein taken in by the diabetic must remain normal and sufficient for growth, development and activity. Too often, once diabetes is diagnosed, and despite the fact that the patient is on insulin, the poor soul is given a near starvation diet, which can only result in poor diabetic control, loss of weight and a perplexed unhappy and hungry patient.

Although there is no true calorie restriction necessary in the diabetic on insulin, dietary discipline is necessary in other ways, and there are three fundamental rules:

First, all refined carbohydrates, candies, cakes, cookies, chocolates and honey are totally forbidden. These may *only* be used in the prevention or treatment of insulin reactions (hypoglycaemia) and this privilege must not be abused. You are taking a set dose of insulin every day and therefore cannot hope to handle the sudden sharp rise in blood sugar that will be precipitated by eating concentrated glucose in the form of refined sugar. In non-diabetics, the intake of refined sugar causes a massive release of insulin which will rapidly convert the load of excess glucose to fat, thereby maintaining a normal blood sugar. By the very nature of the disorder, the diabetic cannot do this, and taking sugar will therefore invariably result in a loss of diabetic control with large fluctuations in blood sugar. A set number of factory workers cannot hope to cope with an unexpected excess of goods suddenly dumped on the factory floor. This can only result in a backlog of unprocessed material which will jam the workbenches of the factory. High blood sugar levels, or large fluctuations in blood sugar can be dangerous in the long term. This is discussed in Chapter 6.

Second, it is essential to eat frequently. In addition to three normal meals, the insulin-requiring diabetic *must* eat regular snacks between meals. In essence, you should eat breakfast, a light mid-morning snack, lunch, a mid-afternoon snack, supper and, most important, a snack before bedtime. This does not imply that you must eat excessively, as the between-meal snacks can be light (for example, cheese and biscuits or a portion of fruit) and can be taken out of the calories normally consumed at the main meal. It is also important that the meals be taken at approximately the same time every day. The injected insulin is acting constantly throughout the day and night, and the blood insulin level cannot drop to low levels between meals, as happens in non-diabetics. Therefore, if you allow many hours to lapse between meals the continuing action of insulin on the blood sugar will result in the sugar dropping too low and insulin (hypoglycaemic or low-sugar) reactions will occur (see Chapter 4). This is particularly likely to happen in the early hours of the morning if the late-night snack is omitted, since the usual time period from supper to breakfast is a long one. If you do not eat regularly, and despite this, do not become hypoglycaemic, this must imply that your blood sugar was too high to start with, suggesting that the insulin dosage is too little. Because of the pressures of day-to-day living, rushing to work, long business meetings and the slow crawl home in the evening traffic, many people develop the habit of eating once, or maybe twice a day, and the meal commonly skipped is breakfast, and often lunch. In general, this is not healthy, and for a diabetic such a practice can be lethal. Far better to pull a crumpled cheese sandwich from your pocket during a mid-morning meeting with the boss than to collapse into a sweating, confused heap and need to be carried out and given sugar. And a forgotten mid-afternoon snack can so easily lead to an inability to concentrate or a period of confusion on the way home in all that traffic!

Third, the total calories taken and the proportions of carbohydrate, protein and fat in each meal should remain relatively constant. This means that you cannot allow yourself to have a four course meal on one night and then grab a sandwich or light snack for supper the following night. The insulin dose remains the same day by day and is balanced according to the food intake. If the calorie and carbohydrate intake varies greatly day-by-day, it becomes impossible to calculate a stable insulin dose to keep the blood sugar constant. For reasons discussed further in Chapter 4, it is impractical and unsafe to manipulate your own insulin dosage daily. It is often difficult for the untrained person to assess equivalent food intakes in different meals, allowing for wide variation in diet. Vast differences can occur in patients trying to keep their dietary intake constant, and one study concerning young patients on unmeasured diets was very instructive. It showed that unbeknown to the patients, their dietary intake varied between 1500 and 4000 calories per day, although they believed they were keeping their dietary intake constant. For this reason, a dietician should be consulted to work out a constant diet. There are many ways of doing this, but I believe that the 'exchange method' of meal planning is probably the best and easiest. Foods are divided into various groups or 'exchange lists'. Each food on the list contains about the same amount of starch, fat and protein as other foods on the list. You are instructed as to the number of exchanges to take from the various lists for the three main meals and the between-meal snacks, depending on your individual requirements. Without much effort you will soon learn the common foods on the exchange lists so that meals can be taken without the bother of consulting pages of diets, or of having to carry a little set of scales to the boss's house when you are invited there for dinner.

In summary then, there are three cardinal rules regarding the diet of the diabetic on insulin:

(1) No sugar.

(2) Three regular meals with three between-meal snacks daily.

(3) The same amount of calories and type of food at the same time every day.

Maturity onset diabetes

As already stated, most maturity onset diabetics are overweight and the most important factor in achieving and maintaining control of blood sugar is weight reduction. Thereafter, the mainstay of the diet is calorie restriction. Firstly, all refined sugars, sweets, cookies and chocolates must be totally avoided. The calories must then be reduced sufficiently to initiate, achieve and maintain adequate weight loss. As a rough and ready rule, it can be said that the calories required can be calculated as:

The individual's ideal body weight (in pounds) X 10. For example a woman weighing 190 lbs who should weigh 120 lbs has a correct dietary intake of 120 X 10 or 1200 calories per day. Once the calories have been calculated and limited accordingly, and once sugar has been eliminated from the diet, it is not really important what proportions of fat, carbohydrate or protein are taken to make up that calories intake as long as there is a healthy balanced diet, excess animal fat is avoided, and three meals per day are eaten. A certain amount of starch and fruit is allowed in the diet, and it is not necessary to exclude them completely.

Within days after starting such a diet, and even before any significant weight loss has occurred, the blood sugar levels will start dropping and diabetic control will improve. Once enough weight has been lost, all evidence of diabetes may disappear and blood glucose levels may be completely normal. This does *not* mean that the diabetes is cured, however. It simply means that it has been controlled by diet. As soon as the diet is disregarded and sugar or too much starch is eaten, or weight is regained, the blood sugar will again rise and the diabetes will again manifest itself. It is therefore most important to realize that the dietary restrictions introduced are life-long, so that you must develop permanent new dietary habits. Unfortunately, as a maturity onset diabetic, you have no alternative. Tablets for diabetes should only be used to reduce the blood sugar if, despite dieting, the diabetes remains uncontrolled. There is no way for diet to be replaced by taking tablets, and the fact that you may be taking tablets for diabetes does not exempt you from the diet. For the same reason, the practice of 'taking an extra tablet' before going out for a meal or when you think you are going to break your diet is strongly discouraged.

In summary, the only way the maturity onset diabetic will remain controlled and healthy is by correct dietary habits and weight loss. There is no alternative and none should be tried. Tablets for reducing blood sugar are only used in individual patients who are not adequately controlled on diet alone and yet are not severely diabetic enough to warrant treatment with insulin. Tablets are no substitute for dietary control. A small percentage of patients may have maturity onset diabetes without being overweight. In these patients the basic principles of diet remain the same. However, the calorie intake may not need to be as restricted so that the patient is encouraged to maintain his weight rather than to lose weight.

### Additional general principles of diet for all diabetics

A question frequently asked by diabetics is whether or not alcohol is allowed. As a general principle alcohol is to be avoided. In the first place alcohol is itself a high calorie food so that alcoholic beverages automatically increase the calorie consumption. This is undesirable in maturity onset diabetics and unnecessary in diabetics on insulin. Alcohol is rapidly utilized for energy in preference to glucose in the blood so that, when taken with food, the blood sugar may be elevated disproportionately after the meal, resulting in loss of diabetic control. On the other hand, if alcohol is taken without eating, it is broken down by the liver as a priority. While this is occurring, the liver is unable to release its stored glucose into the blood so that alcohol taken without food can precipitate severe low sugar (hypoglycaemic) reactions. Therefore, particularly in the diabetic on insulin, alcohol can have a variable effect by either increasing or decreasing the blood sugar levels and the effect is not always predictable. One young man, a diabetic on insulin, proved extremely difficult to control. He complained of frequently awakening in the morning 'full of sugar and ketones' to the extent that he was often nauseous and short of breath. Yet, on the same dose of insulin, he was admitted to hospital three or four times a month in deep hypoglycaemic coma. This went on for months and rational management of this fellow seemed impossible – until one day his wife mentioned that his alcohol intake was perhaps excessive, something he had consistently denied. On being questioned, however, he finally admitted to finishing a half-bottle or bottle of vodka most evenings. After prolonged discussions, he was persuaded to give up drinking alcohol. Since then, 2 years ago, he has not been in hospital once and his overall diabetic control has remained satisfactory. Having said all this, if a diabetic insists on having an occasional social drink, the only alcohol which should be allowed is a small amount of whisky or Bourbon, an occasional 'light' low calorie beer or a glass of dry white wine. Red, sweet or 'heavy' wines, standard beer or white spirits should be avoided. Obviously any 'mixers' used must be glucose free (such as soda or tonic water) and the alcohol allowed must be taken only occasionally and in small amounts.

Much has been written recently about the effects of dietary roughage. Not only can constipation be avoided by diets high in bulk, but it has been suggested that high bulk foods may in fact result in increased ease of diabetic control and reduction of blood sugar levels. Therefore, where possible, roughage should be encouraged. For instance, wholewheat bread is preferable to refined bread, and bran breakfast cereals and fresh fruit and vegetables are recommended. Much research is at present underway into the type and quantity of roughage that is ideal, and no doubt the answer to this will soon emerge.

Another question frequently asked is on the advisability of sugar substitutes. One of the common misconceptions is that honey is healthy for the diabetic. In fact, while honey may contain vitamins and important trace elements, it is also the only form of refined carbohydrate found in nature. Therefore, honey is as undesirable and dangerous for any diabetic as is sugar, and should be totally avoided. In general, it is best for you to train yourself to do without any sweetening. However, artificial sweeteners can be used in moderation by the diabetic. Although some doubt has recently been thrown on the longterm use of artificial sweeteners in high dosage, I believe that used in moderation these substances are probably harmless and they are certainly preferable to the use of sugar itself. The modern diabetic is far more fortunate than his counterpart of years gone by. A large variety of bought foods are now sweetened artificially, including fruit juice extracts, sodas, canned fruit, candies and chocolates. There is one snag, however. Many substances are artificially sweetened with sorbitol. This is a naturally occurring substitute, which, although not sugar, contains as many calories as does sugar. Therefore, sorbitol-sweetened foods will not directly affect diabetic control but will increase the calorie intake. For this reason, sorbitol-sweetened foods may be taken in moderation by diabetics on insulin but should be avoided by diabetics needing to lose weight, such as maturity onset diabetics on calorie restricted diets.

As previously mentioned, diabetics are prone to diseases of their large blood vessels, and therefore as a basic principle, it is advisable to keep a diet low in animal fat. In place of butter you should use a high polyunsaturated fat margarine. These are usually clearly marked and as a general rule soft or 'tub' margarines are low in animal fat. Skimmed milk should be used in place of full cream milk and fatty meats, bacon and eggs should be avoided. Sunflower seed or maize oil should be used for cooking and for salad dressing, if allowed by the doctor.

Finally, it must be remembered that many medicines may contain sugar. In particular, most cough mixtures contain a significant amount of glucose and any diabetic should check with the pharmacist before taking cough remedies as there are some sugar-free cough mixtures made exclusively for diabetics.

# Chapter Four

## Insulin and its use in diabetes

Insulin is a hormone produced by cells in the pancreas. These cells are known as beta-cells and are found in clumps, called the Islets of Langerhans. In the non-diabetic individual, insulin is secreted by these beta-cells in response to many stimuli, the most powerful being the blood glucose level. Thus, as the blood glucose concentration rises, more insulin is produced which then brings down the blood glucose level. In this way, the normal blood sugar is controlled in a very narrow range. Obviously, the blood insulin level varies greatly from minute to minute and from hour to hour, depending upon the body's food and sugar intake and degree of activity, amongst other factors. The diabetic, of course, cannot regulate the blood sugar level adequately because he is unable to produce insulin, and if the insulin deficiency is severe enough, it is often necessary to give the patient insulin.

Some diabetics are afraid of 'going onto insulin' because they are afraid of injecting themselves, frightened of living with dependance upon an injection, or simply unsure of the implications. Often the patient feels that insulin means his diabetes is 'severe' and he will therefore psychologically reject the concept of insulin. In fact, the only dangerous diabetes is uncontrolled diabetes, so it is better by far to be controlled on insulin rather than uncontrolled without it. Many people, too, are frightened by anecdotes concerning insulin injections and about the possibilities of low-sugar reactions (hypoglycaemia, insulin shock). Provided the use of insulin is understood, the injections are correctly administered, the doses kept correct, and the patient eats in the correct manner (see previous chapter) there is no danger or mystique in being on insulin.

## Hypoglycaemia

The single biggest problem is the possibility of hypoglycaemic (low sugar) reactions. This happens when too much insulin is injected or too little food eaten. The insulin causes the blood sugar to drop too low. This causes the body to push out many other hormones in an attempt to raise the blood sugar, one of them being adrenalin. This results in the patient feeling strange and often hungry with perspiration, palpitations, headache, shakes and weakness, nervousness, difficulty in concentrating and double or blurred vision. If the blood sugar is not immediately raised by eating, the second state is reached where the brain becomes unable to function, resulting in confusion, aggression, drowsiness and finally coma. Hypoglycaemia is not always dramatic and, particularly in children, may show as irritability, moodiness or temper tantrums. A young executive, who had been diabetic for many years, was always a soft-spoken placid gentleman. However on rare occasions he turned aggressive and unreasonable, often assaulting and beating his wife. He was so ashamed of these episodes that he never told anyone, including his doctor. His wife, respecting his wishes, also kept this problem a secret. One day, however, he developed one of his 'spells' while out visiting, and assaulted his host's wife with no provocation. Only then did he agree to seek medical help. Surprisingly, as it turned out, he was unaware that the episodes were being precipitated by hypoglycaemia. A minor adjustment in insulin dose and diet were made and he is now a model husband, father and friend. Another young diabetic, after being on insulin for one year, started having repeated blackouts and on two occasions this happened while driving, causing extensive damage to his car although he fortunately escaped unscathed. His family practitioner, suspecting hypoglycaemia, started reducing his insulin dosage. The blackouts continued although the insulin was decreased more and more until the poor fellow was completely uncontrolled with high blood sugars and all the symptoms of diabetes. Despite this his blackouts still persisted. At that stage it was apparent that another cause of blackouts should be considered, and after some tests the patient was found to have epilepsy, unrelated to his diabetes. Once treated for his epilepsy, the blackouts ceased, his insulin dose was adjusted and he has now been well for several years.

It is essential that you learn to recognize the early warning signs of hypoglycaemia, which may vary from person to person; once the signs are recognized, the person can easily recover in a few minutes by eating a little starchy food such as a biscuit, a slice of apple, or a small lump of sugar, chocolate or glucose candy. All diabetics on insulin should carry with them lumps of sugar, a bar of chocolate, or glucose sweets. If a reaction is suspected, there must be no delay in eating this, but the privilege must not be abused. It is essential that members of the family and close friends become familiar with the signs of an insulin reaction so that they can assist by administering sugar rapidly if the need arises.

Glucagon is another hormone which combats hypoglycaemia and raises the blood glucose level. It antagonizes the action of insulin and raises the blood glucose level by releasing stored glucose from the liver. If, as a diabetic on insulin, you are prone to unexpected hypoglycaemic reactions, glucagon should be stored at home and a member of the family should be taught its use. Usually, glucagon is available in a single-dose kit comprising of a vial containing 1 mg dry powdered glucagon and another vial containing 1 ml of diluting fluid. Mix the glucagon as follows:

Prepare an insulin syringe and remove the protective caps from the vials of dry powder and diluting fluid. Then insert the needle into the vial of diluting fluid and withdraw all the fluid. Then insert the needle into the vial containing the glucagon and inject all the fluid. With the needle still in the vial, shake gently until all the powder is dissolved. The glucagon can then be injected into the front of the thigh or the side of the arm. Following the injection, the blood glucose level will rise but the elevation of blood glucose following glucagon is only temporary, so you must always eat when you regain consciousness.

No patient should be denied the benefit of insulin if other methods of treatment are ineffective. Insulin has several advantages – it meets the specific body lack, the dose may be graded for the individual, and in the correct dose it will always lower the blood sugar level. Insulin works!

Types of insulin

Insulin cannot yet be manufactured in the laboratory and it is obtained by extraction from the pancreas of animals. The two animals used in all commercial insulin are either cattle or pigs, so that the insulin may be either beef or pork in origin. Both these insulins are very similar to human insulin and work very well in diabetics, but pork insulin resembles human insulin more closely than does beef insulin. However, beef insulin is more abundant and easier to obtain, so that the majority of insulins available are either beef insulins or a mixture of beef and pork insulins. There are many kinds of insulin available in most countries. Each insulin has different lengths of action and different advantages and disadvantages, so that it is a good idea for you to know something about the action of the insulin you are using.

Some of the important actions of the more commonly used insulins are listed in Table 1. Usually, insulins come in two strengths, 40 units per cc and 80 units per cc, but in the USA the concentration has been standardized to a single strength, 100 units per cc. Apart from the insulins listed in Table 1, there are several newer insulins available in some countries. These are the monocomponent or 'single-peak' insulins, and in essence these are highly purified pig insulins of particular use in patients who are allergic to or resistant to insulin. Often, when a switch is made from the usual insulins to the monocomponent insulins, the dose required can drop quite dramatically, and the higher the initial insulin dose, the more likely it is to decrease. One patient, who was taking 360 units of lente

**Table 1 Characteristics of the more commonly available insulins**

| Type | Appearance | Duration of action (hours) | No. of injections per day |
|---|---|---|---|
| **Rapid** | | | |
| Regular (crystalline, soluble, BP) | Clear | 4–6 | two, three, four |
| Semilente | Turbid | 6–8 | two |
| **Intermediate** | | | |
| Globin | Clear | 19–24 | one or two |
| Rapitard | Turbid | 12–18 | one or two |
| N.P.H. (isophane) | Turbid | 18–24+ | one or two |
| Lente | Turbid | 18–24+ | one or two |
| **Slow** | | | |
| Protamine zinc | Turbid | 36+ | one |
| Ultralente | Turbid | 24–36 | one |

insulin daily, without good diabetic control, was finally very well controlled on 32 units of monocomponent insulin daily. Although the drop in insulin requirements on monocomponent insulin is seldom as dramatic as this, you should nevertheless remember that if you are changed to these insulins you should beware of possible hypoglycaemias.

The type and dose of insulin required is a choice made by the doctor, as is the question of whether there should be one or two injections per day. Often you can manage good diabetic control on one injection per day, which is of course more convenient. However at certain critical times of physical, hormonal and emotional change two injections a day become essential. Thus, at the onset of puberty and for most of the teenage years, as well as during pregnancy, the majority of diabetics need to inject themselves twice a day. A 13-year-old girl who had been diabetic for 4 years was seen because of gradual loss of diabetic control over the past months. She was

31

on one injection per day. At the first mention of going on to two injections, she burst into hysterical crying and sobbing and refused to even consider the option. Unfortunately, although she was generally a delightful child she was excessively spoiled by her parents. They, instead of insisting on obeying the doctor's orders, tended to support their distraught daughter so that she has remained on her one injection per day. This was three years ago, and over this time her diabetic control has been consistently poor, with frequent hypoglycaemic reactions alternating with periods of extremely high blood sugars. This attractive, bright child is courting disaster and the damage her parents have allowed her to inflict on herself will be irreversible.

There is a tendency for some diabetics, particularly when recently diagnosed, to become very concerned over the actual amount of insulin they are taking. One has frequent arguments every time the dose has to be increased by a few units. I know of one 19-year-old girl, for instance, who steadfastly refuses to increase her daily insulin dose above 25 units, and in fact considers it a major achievement if she can reduce by 1 or 2 units for a few days. This, of course, is a rather ridiculous attitude since once you are injecting yourself, you might as well use enough insulin to bring the blood sugar down.

It is important to remember that the non-diabetic adult produces the equivalent of about 60–70 units of insulin per day from his pancreas. Therefore, doses of up to and even over 70 units per day are not uncommon or excessive, and the dose of insulin is only considered to be 'large' when it is over 100 units per day.

A patient requiring insulin for the first time should be controlled in hospital, initially on three or four injections of regular insulin daily. Not only does this allow your doctor to establish the correct insulin dose and 'get to know' your diabetes, but it also allows you to become educated in the use of insulin, insulin techniques and dietary adjustments. Once this has been achieved, a finer and more perfect diabetic control can be obtained with minor changes in insulin dosage at home. When you have been on insulin for some months, you may learn to adjust your insulin to some degree yourself, but several rules must be observed in this regard:

(1) Never alter the dose by more than 2–4 units at a time unless otherwise specified by your doctor.

(2) Never alter the dose more than once every three days as it takes several days to stabilize on a new dose, and because of this –

(3) Wait at least 48 hours after a change in dosage before assessing the response of diabetic control to that change in dosage. By that time, the general pattern of the results of urine testing can be assessed. These patterns and trends are most easily and conveniently seen when the results of tests are tabulated, preferably in a note book ruled for that purpose.

Technique of insulin injection

Several types of syringes are available for injecting insulin. These include glass syringes which are stored in glass containers containing spirits; plastic sterile disposable syringes, or automatic syringes. There is little difference between these various forms but generally, the disposable plastic syringes are preferred, as they tend to be more accurate, more sterile and less trouble than the glass syringes.

It is important to maintain absolute cleanliness at all times throughout the injection. Wash your hands with soap and water and dry them on a clean towel before starting. At this time, the syringe can be removed from the packet (if a disposable syringe is being used), or from the spirits (if a glass syringe is being used). In the latter instance remember that insulin is destroyed by spirits, so that the syringe and needle must be washed out with clean running water from the mains tap or with cool boiled water. Squirt the water in and out through the needle and then empty the syringe of water by squirting out several times. No spirit whatsoever must be allowed to get into the insulin bottle.

33

Alternatively, the syringe and needle may be dismantled and boiled each time they are used. Take the syringe to pieces, place it in warm water, heat to boiling and keep boiling for two minutes. Allow to cool and then reassemble.

Insulin needs to be shaken, so that the bottle must be turned upside down repeatedly for a minute, but must not be

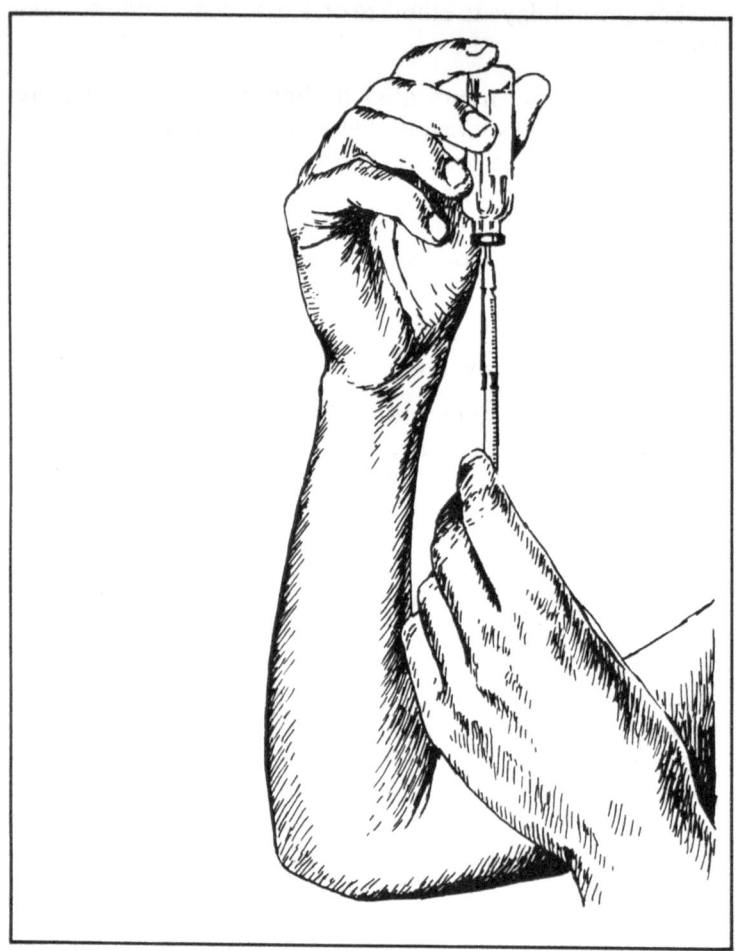

**Figure 5a**

shaken more violently. Paint the top of the rubber cap of the bottle of insulin with a piece of clean cottonwool moistened with either alcohol or ether. Draw back the plunger on the syringe to the mark corresponding to the number of units being withdrawn. Push the needle through the cap injecting the air into the bottle and withdraw the insulin by sucking it into the syringe (Figure 5a). Finish with the syringe containing no air and filled to the required mark with insulin. To withdraw the insulin the point of the needle must be below the level of the insulin and to ensure this the bottle is held cap downwards. When the bottle is nearly empty the needle must not be pushed too far in.

The needle is then withdrawn, and care should be taken that it does not become detached from the syringe. The syringe is then placed on its side on a clean surface, so placed that nothing touches the needle.

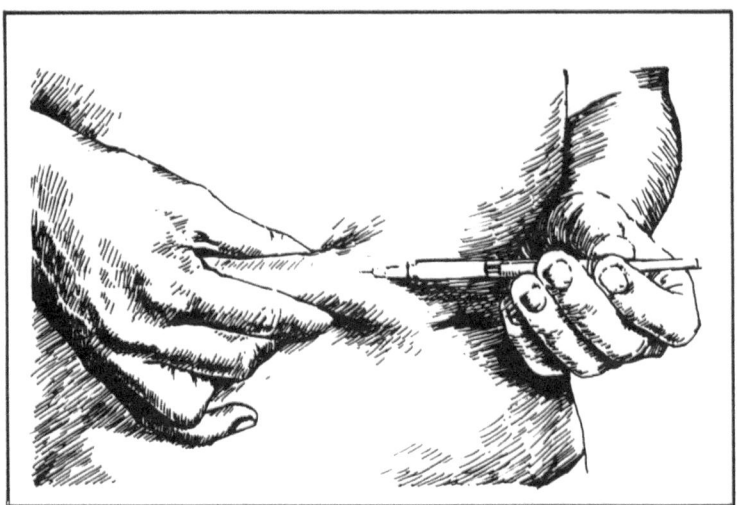

**Figure 5b**

Insulin can be injected anywhere where the skin is loose and there is fat under the skin, but a different place must be

used for each injection. In fact, the site of the injection should be altered every day so that the same place is never used more than once every two weeks. The front of the thigh and the front of the abdomen are good places but the buttocks, sides and upper arms may also be used (Figure 6).

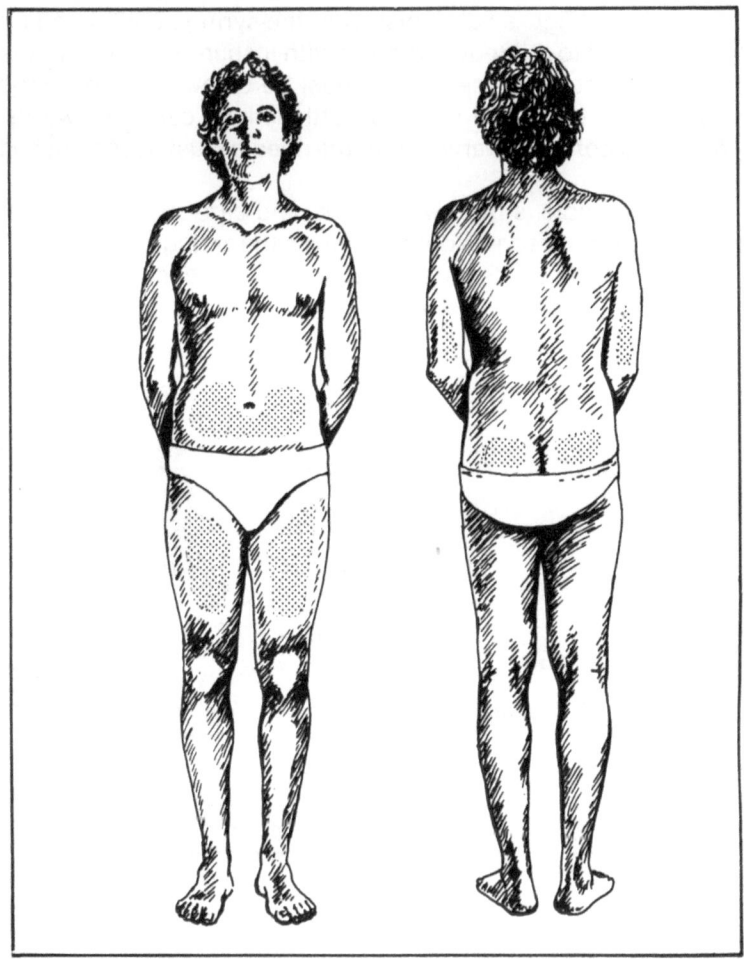

**Figure 6**

Some diabetics get into the very bad habit of injecting in one particular site for a long time. This can result in one of two things. Either, the fat under the skin disappears, causing 'fat atrophy'. This results in an hollowed out appearance at that site – which can mar an otherwise perfect physique or bikini figure. Alternatively, at the site of frequent repeated injection the skin can thicken with scar tissue forming under the skin. Not only does this cause an ugly lump at the site of injection, but insulin injection into this area is inadequately and irregularly absorbed so that diabetic control can suffer. I once saw a patient who had been injecting himself daily for 17 years on one small localized area on the inside of the right thigh. He had developed a large unsightly pendulous growth of scar tissue at that site, which resembled a tumour. The skin was so tough over this growth that two or three needles often snapped before he was able to get his insulin injected. He was requiring at least five times as much insulin as he subsequently needed when he was taught to inject correctly, because of failure of absorption from this scarred site. His only reason for having developed this technique was that the injection had become completely painless because of the scar tissue. He eventually required plastic surgery to remove the unsightly lump. Insulin injections, given properly with constant altering of the site of the injection, should result in no outward signs of the injection whatsoever.

The selected site is rubbed with a piece of cottonwool wet with ether, alcohol or weak tincture of iodine. The skin is then taken up in the fold in the fingers of the left hand and with the right hand the needle is pushed into the fold through the clean site (Figure 5b). The syringe should be held nearly parallel to the skin and the needle pushed in steadily, nearly up to the butt. Do not jab as it hurts more. However, never push the needle right home as occasionally the needle can break at the butt and as long as the needle is not pushed right in, it will be quite easily pulled out if it breaks off at the butt. The tip of the needle should now feel loose in the soft tissue under the skin. Force the insulin in, withdrawing the needle as you do so, so that all the insulin is not left in the same spot. Withdraw the needle, and press the spot with the wool. After half a minute massage the site of the injection to disperse the insulin.

If a plastic disposable syringe has been used it is now discarded. A glass syringe is rinsed out with water and emptied. Spirits are then sucked up into the needle several times and the syringe is returned to the container containing the spirits.

If, after the insulin injection, 'bumps' develop in the skin, it suggests that the insulin has not been injected deeply enough into the fatty tissue under the skin. Alternatively, if the injection is painful with frequent bruising you may be injecting the insulin too deeply.

Irrespective of which insulin is being used it should be taken not more than 20 minutes before a meal. It is usually taken before breakfast and if a second injection is required, this is usually taken before the evening meal.

Mixing insulins

Often, in order to obtain better diabetic control, it becomes necessary to mix an intermediate-acting or long-acting insulin with a shorter-acting insulin. Do not attempt to mix insulin preparations in the bottle. This is best done in the following way (Figure 7):

(1) Inject an amount of air equal to the dose of intermediate- or long-acting insulin into that insulin bottle (bottle A). Withdraw the *empty* syringe at this time without removing any insulin.

(2) Putting the previous bottle aside, inject an amount of air equal to the desired dose of short-acting insulin into that insulin bottle (bottle B) and remove the proper amount of regular insulin, in the normal way.

(3) Return to the first insulin bottle, insert the needle and withdraw the correct amount of the insulin. This final amount in the syringe is the sum of the short- and long-acting insulins giving the correct total measured dose.

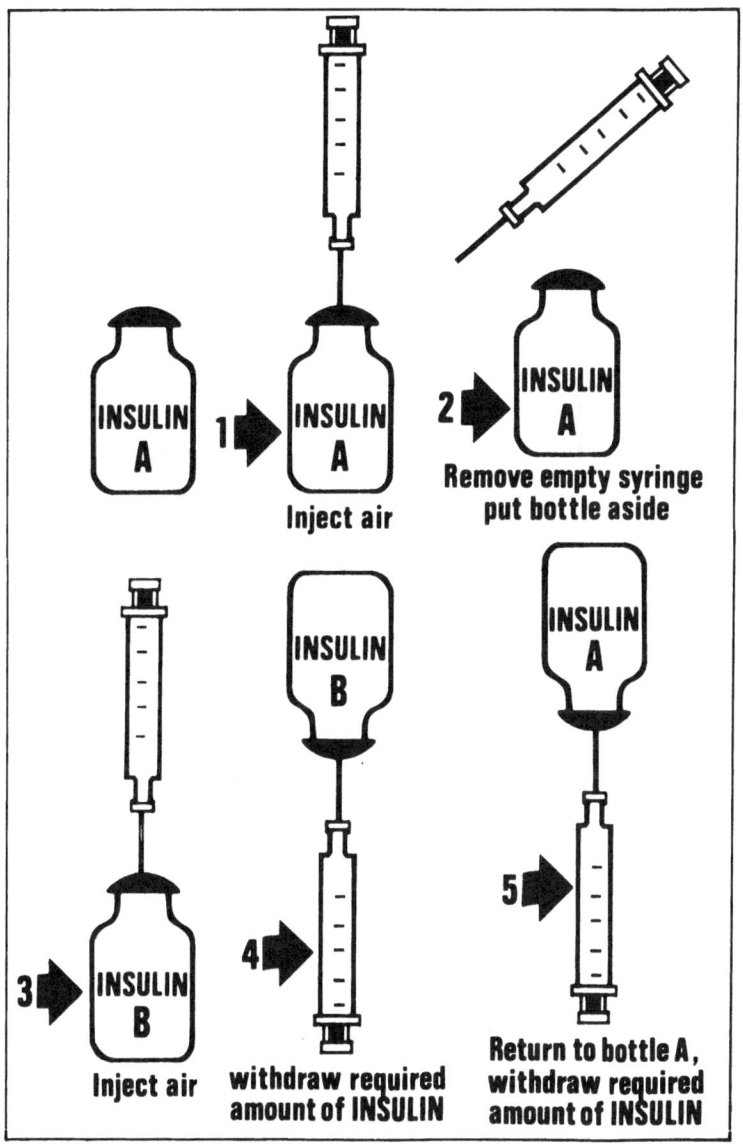

**Figure 7**

Although this technique may sound complicated, you will soon become adept at this procedure and have no trouble with the technique.

Sick days

Illnesses probably cause the greatest problems and uncertainties for the diabetic on insulin. The most serious mistake that can be made is to decrease or omit the insulin because you feel you are unable to eat. During such a period, because of the body's response to the stress of the illness, even the usual dose of insulin may not be sufficient. With illness, you may require *more* rather than less insulin, and this is even more true when the urine tests show large amounts of sugar, particularly if this is accompanied by acetone. If you are very ill, particularly with a temperature, it may be necessary to take regular insulin every few hours until the urine tests improve. The amount of regular insulin needed will vary from diabetic to diabetic, depending on the daily insulin dosage, and initially this should be checked with your doctor. Soon, however, you will learn to make this adjustment yourself. As a general rule, you can add 20% of your usual daily dose, as regular insulin, to the daily dose. This dose of regular insulin can be spread out up to two or three times during the day. Neglecting to give yourself your insulin because you do not feel well enough to eat is the surest way of landing in hospital in diabetic coma.

Testing the urine

Every diabetic should test his urine routinely. Many years ago, this could only be done by tasting the urine. There is a rather quaint story about a professor of medicine who used to insist that all his medical students tasted a diabetic patient's urine by dipping a finger into a glass of the urine and licking the finger. Of course, his students were not too happy about this, so the teacher would set the scene by first doing it himself. However, the crafty old fellow would dip his index finger into the urine and then, with great aplomb, lick his middle finger. Of course, none of the students noticed this and they would then file up to the urine glass for their 'taste' – after all, if the professor could do it, then they must too! Many years went by before a particularly observant student spotted the trick and spoiled the game. Fortunately, medicine has advanced and there are now several different methods available for testing urine sugar levels.

The frequency of urine testing depends upon the severity of the diabetes and the type of treatment. In very mild maturity onset diabetics, controlled on diet alone, it may suffice to test once every two or three days but as a general rule diabetics not on insulin should test their urine once daily, about two hours after the main meal. Since most people eat their main meal at night, this usually means testing at bedtime. As long as the specimen is free of sugar no further tests are necessary, but should there be sugar in the urine, a second test should be carried out the following morning before breakfast. Persistent sugar in the urine in significant amounts over several days is a reason to contact the doctor.

A diabetic on insulin should test his urine at least twice a day, the best time for testing being in the morning, before breakfast and again two hours after the evening meal, which is usually the main meal. This will give a urine sugar reading in the fasting state (before breakfast) and also when the blood sugar should be at its highest (after the main meal). Further tests may be necessary in some diabetics and these can be done before the midday meal and before the evening meal. Ideally, the diabetic should run blood sugar levels close to normal so that sugar should not appear in the urine. In practice this is very difficult to achieve, so that if a small amount of sugar is seen at times, particularly if this is after the main meal, it should not cause much concern. In any event, as previously stated, it is always useful to keep a record of all urine tests in a notebook as this will enable both you and your doctor to assess overall trends in diabetic control. The primary aim is to keep the urine free from sugar, and it is not adequate to try keeping the urine with a small amount of sugar in it, except for a few individual cases. With experience, minor adjustments of insulin dosage can and should be made by yourself according to the rules laid out earlier in this Chapter. If the urine is persistently free of sugar together with two or three unexplained hypoglycaemic reactions, it is an indication to decrease the dose of insulin by two units, whereas persistent sugar in the urine, particularly if there are no hypoglycaemic reactions, suggests that a slight increase in the dose of insulin is necessary. Of course most people, diabetics included, do not relish playing with their urine, and very often diabetics will find an excuse not to test their urine regularly. The commonest rationalization is that you can 'feel' in yourself when your sugar is high, so why test? The answer is simple. Of course you are aware when your sugar is very high or too low, but I defy any diabetic to 'feel' when the blood sugar is slightly elevated. Another story one often hears is that there has not been sugar in the urine for months so it is not worth testing. In this situation, persisting with the urine tests may be the only way you will become aware of a progressive loss of diabetic control before the blood sugar rises high enough to cause symptoms.

In summary, then:

(1) If you are not on insulin, test once daily after the largest meal. If there is sugar in the urine, test again on awakening the following morning.

(2) If you are on insulin, test at least twice a day, on awakening in the morning and again after the main meal.

(3) Repeated hypoglycaemic reactions require reduction in insulin dose by 2 units. Persistent sugar in the urine requires increase in insulin by 2 units.

How to test urine

There are several tablets and tapes commercially available for testing the urine sugar content. Some of these are more accurate than others and some are simpler to use than others; the type most suited to you should be advised by your doctor. These reagents should be kept in a dry cool place, and since they tend to lose accuracy if kept too long, they should be replaced at least every 4-6 months.

When testing the urine, it is essential not to test the first specimen passed, that is, the one which has been in the bladder for some hours. Rather, the bladder should be emptied and 20 minutes later a second specimen obtained and tested. This is a far better reflection of blood glucose at that moment of time.

For any diabetic on insulin it is also important to test for ketones. As previously explained in Figure 3, the ketones are produced when glucose cannot be used for energy. While this may occasionally be due to too little starch in the diet (starvation ketosis), it is much more often due to too little insulin in the bloodstream. Therefore, the presence of ketones together with an excessive amount of sugar in the urine is a danger signal not to be ignored, and your doctor must be contacted immediately. On the other hand, small amounts of ketones present with very little or no sugar in the urine may only mean that there has been insufficient glucose taken in the diet and this may be of little importance. If, however, starvation ketosis persists or is a regular finding this suggests that your diet is deficient in starch and the amount of carbohydrates in the diet must be increased.

At this point it is worth mentioning that the taking of large quantities of vitamin C, a practice often indulged in by many people to prevent the common cold, may cause false positive urine tests. In other words, vitamin C can cause the urine to show a large quantity of sugar when in fact there is no sugar in the urine at all. For this reason, people with diabetes should not take vitamin C.

Finally it is worth remembering that a small proportion of diabetics have renal glycosuria; that is, sugar may pass into the urine even when the blood sugar is low. In these cases, this should have been elicited by your doctor and in this situation obviously urine tests are unreliable indications of control. Similarly, some patients will not spill sugar in the urine even when the blood sugar is high and the same problem applies to these patients. Once again, you will probably have been advised about this by your doctor.

Insulin and exercise

Physical activity and exercise are healthy for all people, diabetics included. The degree of exercise is obviously governed by your general physical condition but as a general rule you should partake of as much exercise as possible. If you are middle-aged, this exercise may consist simply of brisk walking. Don't forget that exercise, apart from the general 'good health' effects, forms as much part of the treatment of diabetes as does insulin or diet; its importance should not be underestimated. In order for exercise to have its maximum effect, patients on insulin should be receiving an amount of insulin sufficient to control the diabetic condition. In general, in the well controlled diabetic, exercise tends to lower the blood sugar level. It will have an effect similar to 'speeding up the conveyer belts' in a factory production line, so that the same number of workers (insulin) will be able to cope with more goods (glucose) faster and more efficiently. Therefore, if unusually severe or prolonged exercise is taken, or irregular exercise is indulged in (such as playing sport twice a week) then extra bread, a fruit, or starch should be eaten just prior to or just after the exercise. If this is not done, a hypoglycaemic reaction may ensue, and this may occur not only at the time of exercise, but even the following day. Many diabetics tend to reduce their dose of insulin on the day that they are planning exercise. This is not a good practice as it will interfere with diabetic control over the entire day for the sake of a few hours exercise. Rather, the insulin dosage should be kept constant and the exercise compensated for by eating more, preferably before the exercise. A sandwich or fruit may be particularly useful in young diabetics in these circumstances. With experience, most diabetics learn to judge just how much extra to eat in order to cope with varying amounts of exercise, so that diabetic control need not be compromised at all.

Storage of insulin

Regular (soluble, crystalline, BP, USP) insulin will maintain its potency for many months even at room temperature. The intermediate- and long-acting insulins (such as lente or N.P.H.), are also quite stable, but less so than the regular type. Consequently, patients should keep a reserve supply in the refrigerator (but not in the deep freeze). For convenience, the bottle in current use may be kept at room temperature. Even if the insulin has to be unavoidably kept at temperatures consistently above 75 °F, the loss of potency is slow enough so that the insulin will probably remain effective for several weeks. Therefore the storing of insulin during travel should present no real problems. It is not usually necessary for thermos bottles or special cooling kits to be used. In most cases, even during summer, the insulin currently being used can be kept safely in a handbag or suitcase. On long trips a supply of insulin, syringes and needles should always be kept in hand luggage and not in a suitcase which is being airfreighted or shipped separately, since loss of luggage or delay in transit may result in the insulin not being available at the necessary time. At best, this can result in a degree of hysteria and a ruined holiday and, at worst, may be dangerous. Recently, one of my patients travelled from London to Los Angeles by air. He kept only one bottle of insulin with him, the rest being packed in his suitcase, which was duly mislaid by the airline. Unfortunately, on the flight he dropped and broke his only insulin bottle. He was on a monocomponent insulin, not yet available in the United States of America, so on landing in Los Angeles, he was unable to replace his insulin at a pharmacist. He eventually had to be hospitalized for restabilization and after 3 days, he terminated his holiday and returned home in disgust. Extra supplies of insulin taken on trips lasting for several weeks, or months, can be stored between layers of clothing in the luggage as this provides insulation from extremes of temperature. During stop-overs, the insulin can be transferred to a refrigerator.

Temporary improvement or disappearance of diabetes

It is not uncommon for someone to have a sudden onset of

severe diabetes, needing insulin for control, and then find that after discharge from the hospital, the insulin dose needs to be reduced progressively. Sometimes it may appear as though insulin is in fact not needed any more. At this stage, you may keep and feel perfectly well on no treatment at all, giving the impression that the diabetes has disappeared. In fact, what is happening is that the diabetes has gone into remission, and the insulin secreting cells of the pancreas have partially recovered and will function for a further short period of time. Invariably, sooner or later the diabetes will then reassert itself and you will need to go back onto insulin. With the second episode, the diabetes remains permanently present. This has been called 'the honeymoon period' of the diabetic. For psychological reasons it is very important to realize that you are by no means cured and that the withdrawal of insulin for a period of time is only a temporary reprieve. This period can last for days, weeks or months but is almost never permanent. During this period of time you should continue testing your urine daily and as soon as sugar reappears in the urine, your doctor should be notified immediately. I know of one patient who, after a short period of time on insulin, was controlled on diet alone for 5½ years before needing insulin again. He is now stabilized on 60 units of insulin and is well controlled.

Reactive hyperglycaemia (Somogyi effect)

Occasionally, particularly in diabetics who have proved difficult to control, one can find the development of the Somogyi effect. This can be described as a situation where, because of a slight excessive dosage of insulin, the blood sugar drops too low, but not low enough to cause real hypoglycaemic symptoms. In response to this low blood sugar, the body pushes out many anti-insulin hormones which causes the blood sugar to be elevated rapidly, so that some hours after this event you may find a large amount of sugar in the urine, even with acetone. The sequence of events is depicted in Figure 8. Very often this happens when the blood sugar drops transiently too low in the early hours of the morning, when you are sleeping and

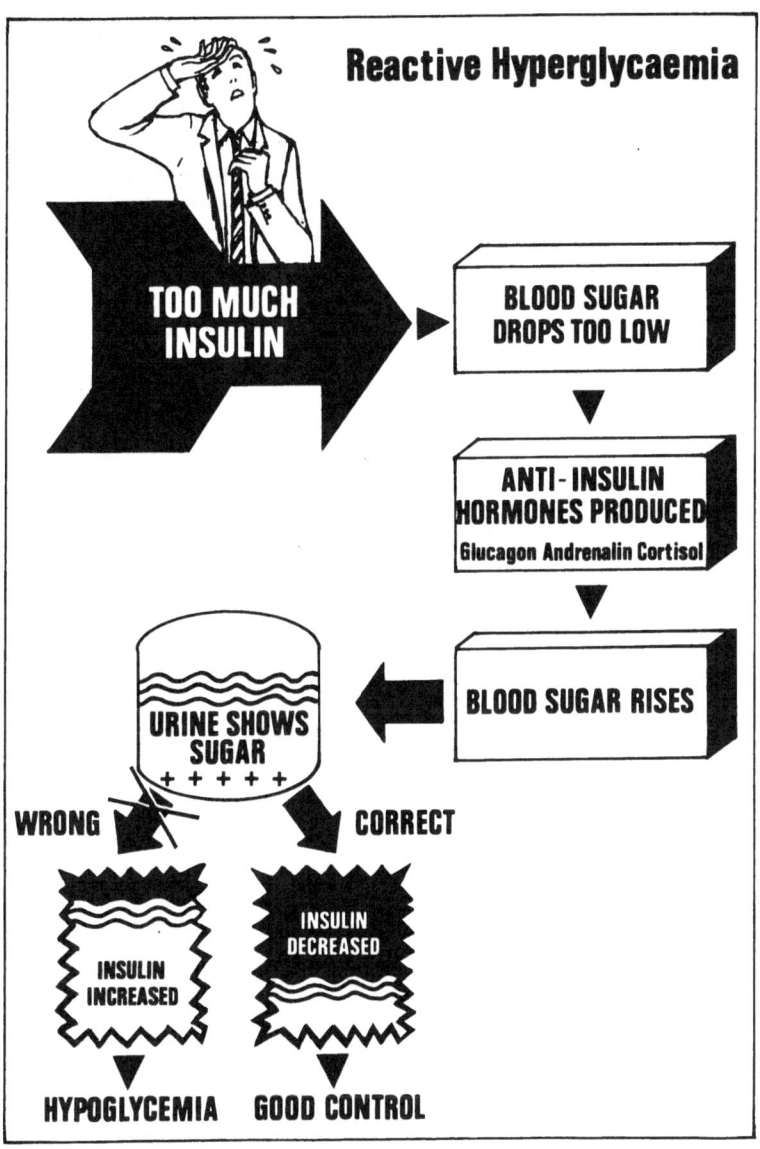

Figure 8

therefore unaware of it, and by the time you wake you find that your urine is full of sugar. The tendency would therefore be to increase the insulin dosage and this will then result in a severe hypoglycaemic reaction in the early hours of the following morning. When this happens, it is often perplexing to the doctor and patient alike. In fact, in these instances, the correct treatment would be, of course, to *reduce* the actual dose of insulin slightly. This phenomenon of reactive hyperglycaemia is difficult to diagnose, even with experience. However, a good indication that it may be occurring would be if there is weight gain in the presence of apparent poor diabetic control. Since poor control is usually associated with weight loss, and consistent low blood sugar levels are frequently associated with weight gain, the paradox of weight gain in the face of apparent poor control must always lead one to suspect the possibility of this phenomenon occurring. If such a situation should arise, it would be unwise for you to attempt to adjust this yourself and the situation should be discussed with your doctor.

Home blood glucose monitoring

In some patients it may be necessary to have frequent estimations of actual blood glucose levels. This may be because you are particularly 'brittle' with frequent wide fluctuations in blood sugar levels, or because urine tests are inaccurate due to an altered renal threshhold for sugar. In pregnancy, also, it is extremely important to maintain perfect diabetic control (see Chapter 7). This can now be achieved by monitoring the blood glucose levels at home, using a drop of blood from a finger prick. Small semiportable machines can be hired or bought to enable a quick fairly accurate blood glucose reading from this drop of blood. If you have problems with diabetic control for any of the above reasons, it would be worthwhile to discuss the possibility of home blood glucose monitoring with your doctor.

# Chapter Five

## *Tablets in the treatment of diabetes*

There are several types of tablets available which are used for diabetes, and some of them have been used for a long time. Often, patients ask why they can't take 'insulin tablets' or 'insulin by mouth'. The first thing to realize is that insulin itself cannot be taken in tablet form as it would be broken down by the acid and enzymes in the stomach, rendering it useless. The available tablets for diabetes work in a different way, either stimulating the pancreas to push out more insulin than it is doing, or by increasing the activity of the available insulin. Therefore, it is obvious that anyone who is going to take these tablets with effect must be capable of producing *some* insulin from their Islets of Langerhans. Juvenile onset diabetics, by the very nature of their disorder, have very little or no insulin and therefore in such cases there is no chance of the diabetes being controlled with tablets. In maturity onset diabetics, on the other hand, there is very often a significant amount of insulin being produced by the pancreas, although not enough to prevent the onset of diabetes. The use of tablets, therefore, is confined to the maturity onset diabetic and tablets are seldom used in juvenile onset diabetics.

The most important point to remember is that the tablets are used only as an addition to diet, *never* in place of it. The diet remains the mainstay of treatment. Frequently, patients say that they take an extra tablet before going out to dinner, as if this will compensate for and justify the expected bout of overeating. This is of course incorrect. There is no compensation for eating incorrectly and an extra tablet will not help one bit. Commonly the excuse is used that because of social or business commitments one cannot help eating the wrong foods. In fact, it must be on rare occasions only that it is truly unavoidable for you to break your diet, and on most occasions the real problem is that you are looking for an excuse. It is amazing how understanding your host and guests can be in this regard. It is not easy to keep to a lifelong diet, doing without the 'good things', but unfortunately it is an absolute necessity to ensure good health. There is no alternative to diet, and certainly tablets are not a substitute. If it should occasionally happen that you weaken and eat incorrectly, you should accept a transient loss of diabetic control rather than increase your tablets.

Tablets are required by maturity onset diabetics, who, despite dieting, remain with high blood sugar levels, though not high enough to require insulin. In these people, the addition of tablets will help bring the diabetes under control.

*The sulphonylureas (Orinase, Tolinase, Dymelor, Rastinon, Diabenese)*

These tablets work by making the pancreas secrete more insulin. However, they have two major disadvantages. The first is that by increasing the blood insulin level, they increase the appetite, making it more difficult to diet. Therefore they promote weight gain rather than weight loss. This unfortunate side effect must be borne in mind if you are an overweight diabetic. Secondly, they can cause the blood sugar to drop too low, causing hypoglycaemic episodes. Also, there is some evidence to suggest that perhaps these tablets promote high blood pressure and even coronary thrombosis. All these facts must be borne in mind and the advantages of the effect on blood sugar weighed up against the possible disadvantages of the drugs before they are prescribed. This is best done by your doctor and there are many many thousands of patients on this treatment and keeping very well on it. One must just remember that all pills have their disadvantages and should not be taken without medical advice and supervision.

## The biguanides (Insoral, Glucophage, DBI-TD)

This is the other major group of drugs used for diabetics. These drugs are no longer in general use in the United States of America, but are still used frequently in many other countries, including the United Kingdom and Europe. They work by making the body tissues more sensitive to the available insulin. These drugs often cause a decreased appetite, do not promote weight gain, and therefore are more suitable for overweight maturity onset diabetics. They also do not cause hypo- glycaemia. However, they do have their adverse effects. Commonly, nausea and diarrhoea can be caused, something which most people do not enjoy. Furthermore, these drugs can be dangerous if kidney function is not normal, if too much alcohol is imbibed (which it should not be, since you are on a diet, remember!) or if the liver is damaged. Once again, then, the same criteria apply as for the other drugs – medical supervision and check-ups are essential. There is no way you can escape your doctor!

Sometimes it is necessary to combine these two groups of drugs for better effect. If this, with diet, does not control the diabetes adequately, the only alternative is insulin, irrespective of age. They say you cannot teach an old dog new tricks, but this is not true with diabetics. Many is the time I have put a patient of 60 or 70 years of age onto insulin, with no problems in adjustment. So often a patient is not controlled despite sincere attempts at dieting and maximum doses of tablets. Month after month, visit after visit, the patient is begged and implored to go onto insulin. 'I am too old, doctor' or 'I couldn't ever inject myself' or 'I have been diabetic for fifteen years and still feel well, so why should I change now?' are the sort of excuses one hears. Finally, after many months, the patient reluctantly agrees to 'give insulin a try'. Three months later, the same patient's only complaint is that he was not put onto insulin many years ago since he feels so much better. If you are not controlled with tablets, do not be afraid of insulin. It is really not difficult to administer and you will feel better and live longer.

# Chapter Six

## Complications of diabetes

Unpleasant as the subject may be, it is important and realistic to mention that diabetics, especially those who have been careless with their diabetic control or their treatment in general, may develop certain complications. These may in time involve many of the organs of the body.

### Diabetes and your heart and circulation

Heart disease is very common in diabetics, particularly maturity onset diabetics, and often the diagnosis of diabetes is only made when an elderly diabetic develops angina or a coronary thrombosis. The increased incidence of heart disease is probably, at least in part, because of the abnormalities in fat metabolism found in uncontrolled diabetics, with the tendency to an elevated blood cholesterol and triglyceride level. The high fat levels cause fat deposits on the walls of the blood vessels. This can result in gradual narrowing of the arteries, until blood can pass through the narrowed vessels only with difficulty. Narrowed vessels, when the walls are damaged by fat, also cause blood to clot so that a thrombosis (clot) can develop in the walls of the arteries, further obstructing the blood supply. This can happen to those arteries supplying blood to the heart muscle itself (the coronary arteries) resulting in a coronary thrombosis and damage to the heart muscle. It can also happen to other major arteries such as those to the brain, causing a stroke, those to the kidneys, causing kidney problems and those arteries to the legs,

**Table 2 Known risk factors in the development of angina and coronary thrombosis**

| Major factors | Contributory factors |
|---|---|
| Smoking | High serum uric acid (gout) |
| High blood fats (cholesterol and triglycerides) | Stress |
| Diabetes | Lack of exercise |
| High blood pressure | Obesity |
| | Family history of coronary thrombosis |

resulting in poor circulation to the legs. Not surprisingly, obesity is also associated with high blood fat levels. Therefore there is a higher incidence of heart and circulatory disturbances in overweight people than is found in normal people. Smoking is yet another major factor in causing these problems (see Table 2). So if you are diabetic and overweight, and smoke, you are playing Russian roulette! What can you do about it? Obviously you can always lose weight and stop smoking – not easy but not impossible – but what about the diabetes? It will not go away and you must live with it, but good diabetic control will control not only the blood sugar levels but will also lower the blood fats, reducing the chances of developing these problems. All the important risk factors have been listed in Table 2, and as you will see, most of them are self-induced and preventable! I had one obese diabetic patient who prided himself on the fact that he consumed one dozen eggs and one pint of milk every day of his life. He also smoked 60 cigarettes per day. Not surprisingly, he had severe angina. After many weeks of persuasion, he promised to mend his ways. He came in one day, very proud of himself, reporting that he had reduced his egg intake to 6 per day and he had reduced his smoking to 40 cigarettes per day. He was shocked and dismayed when I intimated that this was not good enough, and adamantly refused to make any further concessions to 'this nonsense'. Sadly but predictably, he had a coronary thrombosis and died some months later. This sort of patient makes the practice of medicine seem a futile and un-rewarding pastime, but fortunately most patients tend to be more cooperative.

Circulation can also be affected by the narrowing of the small blood vessels in the muscles and skin, not as a result of high blood fats, but due to thickening of the walls of the small vessels themselves. This is probably directly related to a high uncontrolled blood sugar and it can take many years to develop.

Interference with circulation to the legs is of particular significance, since there is often an associated loss of feeling in the feet (discussed later in this Chapter). Therefore, one may damage one's feet without being aware of it or feeling the pain, and ignore the wound. The wound may not heal because of a combination of the diabetes and poor circulation. It can then become infected and the infection may spread. This can result in gangrene of the foot with all its unpleasant consequences. This is the reason we always stress the importance of foot care, particularly if the diabetes has been present for a long time. Most important in this regard, is that any cuts, wounds, or cracks in the skin of the foot, should be immediately treated by a doctor before problems can develop. For the same reason corns and bunions should never be scraped, toenails should not be cut too short, and you should be careful of walking barefoot, particularly where sharp stones are around. Shoes must fit well, and you should avoid blisters from badly-fitting footwear. If the skin of the feet becomes dry or cracked, lanolin cream should be rubbed into the feet twice daily to keep the skin supple. Feet should be looked after; you need them to carry you around for many years to come. There are many horror stories in this regard. One that comes to mind is the sixty-year-old man, diabetic for many years, who developed a swollen big toe the day after standing on a needle. The toe was not particularly painful (because of diminished sensation) and he thought it was probably gout, since he had suffered from gout intermittently for many years. Disregarding one of the fundamental rules of foot care, he therefore chose to 'wait a few days and see' before going to his doctor. Unfortunately, within

48 hours the swelling and pain extended over his entire foot and ankle and by the time he sought medical attention he had a fever, and was septicaemic. After many weeks in hospital he finally went home, having had his leg amputated above the knee. This could all have so easily been avoided by an immediate visit to his doctor when he first stood on the needle.

High blood pressure is very common in diabetics, particularly the maturity onset diabetic. In diabetic patients over the age of 50 years, as many as 41% may have high blood pressure. Since hypertension (high blood pressure) in its own right is considered a major risk factor in the development of a coronary thrombosis and strokes, it stands to reason that in an uncontrolled diabetic, untreated hypertension compounds this probability many times. The crux of the matter is that good control of diabetes and blood fats and treatment of high blood pressure are all essential components towards leading a full healthy and long life. In addition, remember that smoking, unhealthy for anyone, is an absolute disaster for a diabetic.

### Diabetes and the eye

Most diabetics have experienced blurring of vision when their diabetes is uncontrolled. This is temporary and fairly harmless. The explanation is quite simple. When the blood sugar is high, it is converted into another substance called sorbitol, which is stored in many tissues, one of which is the lens of the eye. When the sorbitol content in the lens rises, it pulls fluid into the lens causing swelling of the lens. As the blood sugar drops, the sorbitol is used up and the water passes out of the lens, causing the lens to shrink. This swelling and shrinking of the lens of the eye interferes with vision and can cause fairly marked disturbances and blurring of vision.

More serious than this are the longterm effects of diabetes on the eye, and the greatest fear of most diabetics is the possibility of losing vision. In fact, relatively few diabetics ever become completely blind, probably less than 5%. It is thought that the major factor promoting diabetic eye disease (retinopathy) is the presence of uncontrolled high blood sugar levels.

In the same way as this may cause thickening of the small vessels to the muscles and skin, it can also cause thickening of the small vessels to the retina, with areas of weakness in these blood vessels. Initially, this produces no noticeable effects and may only be seen on routine examination. Sooner or later, however, one of these small vessels may rupture causing bleeding into the eye chamber. If there is little bleeding, it may not interfere with vision, but a large bleed can cause a sudden loss of vision and the larger the bleed the more severe is the eventual impairment of eyesight. These damaged small vessels may also result in the development of new vessels which grow in a haphazard fashion from the back of the eye into the chamber of the eye. Not only are these new vessels more prone to bleeding than normal vessels, but as they grow forward from the back of the eye, they can cause the retina to detatch, resulting in blindness.

For these reasons it is vitally important for every diabetic to have his or her eyes checked by an eye specialist at regular intervals. As a general rule, your eyes should be checked once every two years but if the eye specialist sees or suspects problems, you may be asked to return more frequently.

Areas at the back of the eye which look damaged or new vessels seen growing from the back of the eye, can be treated with photocoagulation. Photocoagulation is, quite simply, a method whereby concentrated light rays or laser rays are aimed at the back of the eye and pinpointed on the troublesome vessels, causing them to clot and shrivel so that they cannot later rupture, bleed, or grow new vessels. This method of treatment is very effective if properly done and as long as the photocoagulation is kept away from the main visual centres of the eye, it does not interfere with eyesight. However, once again prevention is obviously far better than cure and good diabetic control will prevent or delay the onset of this diabetic retinopathy. It has also been suggested that cigarette smoking may hasten the onset of diabetic retinopathy, so here is yet another very good reason not to smoke.

It has long been known that diabetics appear to be more prone to develop cataracts than the general population. A cataract is simply an opacification or milkiness which appears in the lens of the eye, thereby impeding the passage of light into the eye and reducing vision. Once again, cataracts may occur more commonly in diabetics who are uncontrolled than in those who maintain good blood sugar levels. This is particularly true of cataracts developing in young diabetics. Interestingly, it has also been shown that some types of cataracts can improve considerably if the diabetes is properly controlled. If cataracts should develop and become dense enough to impede eyesight significantly, surgery can be performed to remove the lens thereby improving vision quite considerably. This is a very effective operation with good results.

## Diabetes and the kidney

Diabetes can affect the kidney in many ways. It has often been said that diabetics are more likely to get infections of the urinary tract than are non-diabetics. This is not altogether true. In fact, the only diabetic population group that is more prone to urinary tract infections are women over the age of 60 years. All other diabetics have no greater incidence of kidney infections than have non-diabetics, provided the diabetes is under control.

Kidney function can be affected by interference with the circulation to the kidneys, due to the deposition of fat and blood clots along the arterial walls, as described earlier. In addition, the small blood vessels in the kidneys may become thickened and narrowed with uncontrolled diabetes. This can cause the kidneys to lose much of their 'filter' effect so that proteins in large quantities can pass through the kidneys. If the kidney in this way loses too much protein, the protein content of the blood can drop and this can cause swelling of the ankles and face. This is known as the nephrotic syndrome, and when it occurs due to diabetic kidney disease it is referred to as the Kimmelsteil–Wilson syndrome. In this situation, kidney function in itself can become impaired and kidney failure may result. In these cases, testing the urine for glucose becomes unreliable. It should be mentioned that *small* amounts of protein are often passed into the urine by longstanding diabetics and this may be of little significance. On the average, protein is found in the urine about 14 years following the onset of diabetes, and only a small proportion of these patients may go on to develop true kidney problems and possible kidney failure.

A problem that may occur in diabetics, albeit infrequently, is that of diabetic bladder atony. The bladder becomes insensitive so that one is not aware that the bladder is full. This causes the bladder to over-distend and it loses most of its muscle and contraction power. This is due to damage to the nerves that control this function, and results in incomplete emptying of the bladder and stagnation of the urine. The stagnant urine is a perfect place for bacteria to grow and frequent bladder infections can occur.

Diabetes and the nervous system

The nervous system can be affected in many ways by diabetes. Symptoms can occur in any nerve pathway anywhere in the body. They can vary from being mild and just annoying to being very severe. Not infrequently, some diabetics complain of sharp, shooting or lightning pains, usually in their feet. These may be transitory and not very severe or may be so painful as to be incapacitating. Sometimes, this is associated with extreme sensitivity and pain on the soles of the feet. Some patients compare the sensation to 'walking on broken glass', and one patient, a young executive, took to walking on his toes, barefoot, carrying his shoes in his hands whenever possible. This gave him a rather sinister, burglar-like melodramatic appearance which, although he looked amusing, demonstrates the degree of discomfort that can be caused by a painful peripheral neuropathy. This kind of painful neuropathy is usually temporary and is very often associated with poor diabetic control, but may occur during restabilization of a poorly controlled diabetic. Usually, these sort of pains take 6–8 weeks to disappear but may last for up to a year. The one

59

redeeming consolation about this painful neuropathy is that it will eventually go away.

Sometimes a diabetic may develop a numbness or loss of sensation, again usually in the feet but sometimes in the hands, feeling like persistent pins and needles in the affected limbs. Once this develops, it is usually permanent and one must learn to live with it. The major disadvantage of this sort of neuropathy, once one has become used to it, is the fact that pain is not felt in the affected limb. If the feet in particular are involved, you must keep a close look out for possible wounds which can become infected.

Although it is not common, occasionally a diabetic may develop sudden paralysis of any one nerve in any one part of the body. This is known as a mononeuropathy. There may be many reasons for this, and sometimes it may improve and sometimes it may not.

The autonomic (involuntary) nervous system may also be affected by diabetes. This may result in low blood pressure with dizziness on standing, chronic diarrhoea or impotence. Once these symptoms develop, they are usually not reversible. Impotence is often the earliest manifestation of autonomic nervous system involvement, and its implications are discussed further in Chapter 10.

There is one overriding common denominator to all these complications of diabetes; they all develop more frequently, more severely and earlier in the uncontrolled diabetic. The message should be quite clear. Provided proper care is taken, treatment is adhered to and regular check-ups are made, the chance of developing any of these unpleasant side effects of diabetes is greatly diminished.

# Chapter Seven

## *Pregnancy and diabetes*

During pregnancy, many internal changes occur which may promote the development or worsening of the diabetic state. This is not only because of the general stress of pregnancy to the mother, but also because the fetus and placenta produce many hormones which have an anti-insulin effect. This effect can manifest itself in four ways:

(1) Diabetes may occur for the very first time during a pregnancy in a woman who has never been known to be diabetic previously. This may be very mild diabetes or may be severe enough to require insulin. The major feature of this kind of diabetes is that it usually disappears after the child has been delivered, and may reappear only in subsequent pregnancies. This is called *gestational diabetes.* 25% of women who develop this kind of diabetes remain diabetic after childbirth.

(2) Diabetes may have been present in an undetected form prior to the pregnancy, and the pregnancy may then cause the diabetes to become clinically obvious, and it may remain permanently after the delivery of the child.

(3) Known mild diabetics may become more severe so that a woman who has previously been controlled on minimal treatment may require insulin, which may continue permanently.

(4) In the usual situation, the mother is a known diabetic on insulin, and the insulin requirements will be increased

quite considerably throughout the duration of the pregnancy. Soon after the child is born, the insulin dosage should drop back to prepregnancy levels.

The influence of pregnancy upon the course of the diabetes varies as the pregnancy progresses. During the first three months we often notice that the degree of diabetes appears to lessen and the insulin dependent mother may become more sensitive to insulin, so that the insulin dosage drops progressively. The second three months of the pregnancy is characterized by a gradual increase in the severity of the diabetes. During this period the insulin requirement increases and the patient's diabetes becomes more difficult to control. The last three months of the pregnancy is characterized by an even more marked diabetic state and the insulin requirements go even higher. Overall, most diabetic women will need to increase their insulin dose by as much as another two thirds over the prepregnancy dosage during the course of the pregnancy.

During the entire duration of the pregnancy it is extremely important for the mother to keep her diabetes in excellent control. One patient described this as 'walking an insulin tightrope', a very apt description. Persistently high blood sugars can be harmful to the unborn child, whereas repeated hypoglycaemia is both unpleasant and dangerous to the mother. Interestingly, hypoglycaemic attacks in the mother appear to have no ill effects on the fetus.

A critical period in diabetic control occurs at about 12 weeks of pregnancy, when the insulin dose starts to rise. At this time, it may become necessary to admit the expectant mother to a nursing home for restabilization. Diabetics who have been on one injection per day are usually, at this stage, converted to two injections per day for the remainder of the pregnancy in order to attain ideal control of diabetes.

During pregnancy the mother is particularly prone to develop ketones in the blood and urine (see Chapter 1). This may occur even when the blood sugar is itself not too high and may be related to insufficient starch intake to meet the needs of the mother and the child. Therefore the blood and urine should be regularly checked for acetone, and if it is present in the absence of any sugar in the urine, it should be treated by increasing the starch intake in the diet (unrefined starch, not sugar). Another problem that occurs in pregnancy is the frequent occurrence of renal glycosuria; by that is meant that the kidney will tend to filter sugar into the urine at a lower blood sugar level than is normally the case. This of course may result in high urine sugar tests in the face of reasonable blood sugar levels. It is very important to be aware of this phenomenon, as when it occurs the usual urine tests become an inaccurate reflection of what is going on in the blood. In these circumstances the diabetes often has to be controlled by measuring the blood sugar levels frequently.

Furthermore, sugar lost in the urine represents calories lost and therefore, although the pregnant diabetic may be eating an apparently adequate diet, so much sugar may be lost in the urine that the calorie intake may in fact be inadequate. This may result in the development of ketones in the urine. This happened to one of my patients during her first pregnancy. She had been given an excessively calorie-restricted diet in order to avoid excessive weight gain during the pregnancy. As the pregnancy progressed she developed severe renal glycosuria. Her doctor therefore found her to have persistently elevated urine sugar readings with high levels of ketones. She was hurriedly admitted to hospital for restabilization, where she remained for several weeks, during which time a discrepancy between the blood and urine sugar estimations were repeatedly documented. During this time this patient was losing 600–800 calories per day in the urine. Since she was on a 1200 calorie diet, it is not surprising that she was losing weight and feeling ill, as she had an actual intake of only 400–600 calories per day. It is also not surprising that she had a starvation ketosis. Finally, once the problem was realized, her diet was increased to 2000 calories per day, the ketonuria disappeared and her sugars were controlled by repeated blood sugar estimations. She went on to a normal pregnancy with well controlled diabetes and gave birth to a beautiful son some months later. All these factors have to be carefully assessed and the insulin dosage has to be carefully and frequently adjusted.

The last weeks of the pregnancy are particularly hazardous for the unborn child, and because of this it is practice to terminate the pregnancy a few weeks early, at about 36 weeks. Often this is achieved by means of a Caesarean section but occasionally a normal vaginal delivery can be induced. The decision as to which method of delivery should be tried is entirely in the hands of the obstetrician who knows the various advantages and disadvantages of both methods and will take them into account in each individual situation. He will also decide on the exact timing of the delivery, usually by doing repeated blood tests which assess the health and growth rate of the baby. He may also use ultrasound scanning; this is a test where sound waves are passed through the womb (much like radar) and the exact size of the baby can be assessed with complete safety. With these measures available, the obstetrician can decide on the precise moment that the baby should be delivered and the safest method of delivery.

Effect of pregnancy upon the complications of diabetes

If there is no evidence of any diabetic complications (as outlined in Chapter 6) then the pregnancy will not hasten the development of any of these complications. However, any neuropathy which may be present can be intensified by the pregnancy. This is usually temporary and with childbirth, the neuropathy returns to its previous degree. There is no major effect on kidney function, provided that severe diabetic kidney disease is not established before pregnancy. However, diabetics who fall pregnant are more prone to urinary tract infections than the general population, and this should be borne in mind, routinely checked for, and treated if it arises.

The major complication which causes concern in pregnancy is the presence of diabetic eye disease. If there is significant retinopathy present, this can be intensified in pregnancy and is irreversible. Therefore, the one major contraindication for pregnancy in a diabetic is the presence of established retinopathy.

### Effect of diabetes on the course of pregnancy

Before the discovery of insulin, women with diabetes found it extremely difficult to become pregnant. However, today, with adequate treatment of the diabetes, fertility is unimpaired. In fact, if fertility is measured by family size, it has been found that diabetics have larger families than non-diabetics.

Provided the diabetes is well controlled and the woman is in a good state of health without major diabetic complications, there is no increased risk of miscarriage in the pregnant diabetic as compared to the general population.

Once pregnancy is established, if the diabetes is adequately controlled, the course is usually uneventful until the delivery is precipitated by the obstetrician at about 37 weeks. The baby, at birth, tends to be larger and fatter than babies born to non-diabetics. This is due to early excessive fat deposition. There is also a tendency for the baby's blood sugar to drop too low soon after birth. Therefore, whenever possible, a child specialist should be on hand to treat the newborn baby in the first few days.

### Family planning

It is generally accepted that pregnancy and childbirth are less problematical and easier in a younger woman, and most obstetricians would recommend, where practicable, that the first pregnancy should be before the age of 30 years. This applies even more to the woman with diabetes. Not only is the pregnancy and delivery easier and less likely to show complications if the mother is younger, but there is always the chance (however slight) of the onset of diabetic retinopathy or other diabetic vessel disease developing as the years go by. For this reason, it is often recommended that a diabetic woman have her family, say two or three children, as soon after marriage as is practicable and then practice contraception. This is sound advice, although there are many examples of diabetics having families much later in life. One patient, having had diabetes from the age of 10 years, had her first child at 37 years of age, a second child 3 years later and another child at the age of 42 years. All three pregnancies were uneventful and all her children are healthy and well.

Many types of contraception can be considered. Some gynaecologists do not approve of using an intrauterine device (such as the 'loop', Copper T or Copper 7) in diabetics because of the possibility of introducing an infection into the uterus. The contraceptive pill may interfere with diabetic control, but if there are no reasons prohibiting its use other than the diabetes, the 'mini-pill' (low oestrogen content pill) is probably quite safe. Diaphragms and foam pose no special problems in the diabetic, but have a high failure rate, so that unwanted pregnancies may ensue. Many diabetics opt for sterilization after completing their families, or their husbands ask for a vasectomy. This, of course, is the surest way of avoiding further pregnancies but is an irreversible step. There can be no changing your mind later! The best contraceptive method is therefore an individual choice which must be made in conjunction with a knowledgeable gynaecologist.

# Chapter Eight

## *A child with diabetes*

Diabetes is not a common disease in childhood. It is found in only one child in 2500 below the age of 15 years.

Usually, the onset of diabetes is rapid in childhood, the child usually needing urgent hospital admission. Then, within days, weeks or months after treatment, about one third of all the children experience a state of remission where the diabetes appears to improve or even disappear. This can last anything from a few weeks to many months before the diabetes returns, but return it always does. Between the second and the sixth year following the initial onset of diabetes, the total diabetic state develops and becomes permanent.

In diabetes there is interference with the use of glucose and energy, and so one might expect some interference with growth and development. This was certainly the case in the pre-insulin era, but with present day treatment satisfactory adult height is usually achieved in most children with diabetes.

Management of the child with diabetes

The vast majority of children who develop diabetes will need to be controlled on insulin. This must, of course, be combined with dietary management and although such dietary management of the child with diabetes is second in importance to the insulin therapy, it remains an essential part of the treatment. In this regard, it can be extremely difficult to control the diet of a child. Children, particularly the very young, cannot be made to understand the importance of eating regularly, and if they are not hungry, they will tend to miss out meals. Furthermore, they are by the very nature of our society drawn to refined carbohydrates such as candies, soda and cookies. It is extremely difficult to teach a child to voluntarily refrain from these things when attending parties or outings. Nevertheless, this is one restriction which must be insisted upon. A child may also not recognize the onset of hypoglycaemic symptoms and therefore it falls upon the parent to learn to observe early hypoglycaemia in their children by noticing the advent of sweating, tremor, vagueness or other changes.

Parents of children with diabetes face special problems. Their attitude is extremely important, since children sense feelings in the parents which they frequently reflect into their own developing personalities. All the common sense, thoughtful consideration, and careful handling which the parent can muster are required. The parent must remember that the child, despite his diabetes, needs to go through the same stages of development as other children and the single largest mistake which parents of diabetic children make, is to develop an attitude of overprotectiveness. This approach was taken to an extreme by the mother of a 12-year-old diabetic girl who had been diabetic since the age of 7 years. This woman, with all the best intentions, was obsessed with the fear of allowing her daughter to feel 'different' from other children. Not only would she not *allow* her daughter to test her urine (she insisted on doing this herself, only once a day) but she insisted on giving her child the insulin injection and would not even entertain the idea of the girl learning to inject herself. Furthermore, she refused to accept any dietary restriction, permitting the child to eat whatever and whenever she wanted 'like any normal child'. Worse still, all discussions with the doctor had to be conducted with the child out of the room. This sort of pathological overprotectiveness does irreparable harm and I can only fear for this child's eventual psychological adjustment and ability to care for herself when she finally becomes independent (which she must, eventually).

Parents must appreciate that children cannot be regimented in the same way as adults, and therefore diabetic control cannot at best match the ideal. Invariably, there will be times when urine tests become strongly positive and the blood sugar levels become high, but this must not discourage the parent from aiming for the best possible control. At the same time, testing the child's urine too frequently, restraining activity, and denying the child independence will do irreparable harm to his developing personality.

The importance of the family

As far as the child is concerned, he is much more firmly part of the family unit, including the parents and siblings, than is an adult with diabetes. As in any other disease, the mother, the parent most intimately involved with the child, is usually made supervisor of the diabetes. Her own degree of emotional maturity will play a vital part in determining how realistically she can approach her task. Having a sick child, be it from diabetes or any other chronic illness, will result in the mother becoming extremely anxious about that particular child. Very often, the mother may feel that it is her fault that her child has diabetes, and the child may sense this. The resentment which may thus be created can lead to difficulties between them. The child is often treated as though he were entitled to special considerations, over and above the other siblings, because of his illness. Such a distorted emotional approach may cause the child to feel physically defective and unable to cope with the ordinary demands of life. This must be avoided and the parents, particularly the mother, must do all in her power to make the diabetic child feel the equal of the other children in the family. The child should not be made to feel that his regular injections and dietary restrictions set him apart from his family. This can be achieved by the development of a casual but firm approach. Not all parents have the insight into their own behaviour to develop the correct interrelationship with their diabetic child. If problems arise in this regard, it may be extremely worthwhile to seek psychological counselling, particularly if the handling of the illness interferes with the family unity.

At no time should the diabetic child be made to feel 'special' nor for that matter should the non-diabetic siblings be allowed to feel neglected. The healthy siblings may envy the diabetic child who requires special attention and special food and often the envy is mixed with anger. Siblings can sometimes create difficulty for the diabetic child by teasing him or rejecting him. It is therefore very important that the healthy children be actively and openly included in the total treatment programme and in discussions both with the family and with the patient's doctor.

Most children who enter adolescence go through a period of 'adolescent revolt' and the severity of this revolt relates to the degree of exaggerated parental control in the earlier years. If the child is overprotected, when he enters his phase of emotional adolescent revolt, in order to display independence, he will attempt to remove himself from those facets which he has found most binding in childhood. The danger is therefore that the child will reject those things he has been taught are necessary for diabetic control simply because he has learnt them from his parents. In this stage, much damage can be done. In order to prevent this, the parent must start to shift the responsibility of the diabetic control from himself to the child, several years before the adolescent period. Thus when the child enters adolescence he is already responsible for the care of his diabetes and it has become second nature to him. The child is then less likely to discard his diabetic care. By the time the child is 10 years old he should be able to take responsibility for administering his insulin himself, testing his own urine and recording the tests. The child must also learn to be responsible to himself and his physician for control of his diabetes. By the time the child is 12 years old, he should be attending his doctor on his own, while his parents wait in the waiting room.

The diabetic at school

The young diabetic first entering school has special problems because he has to function normally and effectively together with other healthy children who are not subject to the restrictions which have been imposed on him by his diabetes. He may find difficulty in keeping to a proper diet, particularly in taking his mid-morning snack at the right time. Exercise may cause some difficulty since exercise periods are often irregularly scheduled at school, so that the child may find it difficult to find time to eat correctly just prior to, or after, the exercise period. In addition to this, the diabetic child is extremely anxious not to appear different from his healthy classmates. Most of these problems can be overcome if the child is well educated into the basic fundamentals of his diabetes and understands the inter-relationships between food, insulin and exercise. Often, the co-operation, understanding and assistance of the teacher is required. For this reason, parents of a diabetic child should make an effort to meet the teacher on a personal basis, discuss the problems; and ascertain that the teacher understands the basic principles of diabetes. It is extremely important for the child to learn to recognize the early signs of hypoglycaemia as this can often occur during school hours. If there is some difficulty in the child recognizing this, the teacher should be aware of the impending signs and should have a glucose substance available.

Camps for diabetic children

Over the past years, the majority of diabetic associations in most countries in the world have developed 'diabetic camps'. These are extremely useful innovations and can be an important part of the necessary education process. They teach the children how to look after themselves and allow the children to gradually attain self sufficiency and independence. One of the most important advantages of these camps is that the child learns that he is not really different from other healthy children.

# Chapter Nine

## *General directives in management*

It must be already apparent that it is essential for a diabetic to establish a close rapport with his doctor. You obviously need a doctor who is frank with you and who can be contacted with ease in times of an emergency. Similarly, you must be truthful to yourself and your doctor. It is not unusual for a patient to ignore all instructions from one visit to the next and not bother to test his urine or keep to any sort of diet, only to discipline himself strictly for 2 or 3 days before the next visit to the doctor, so that his blood sugar levels, when checked, appear well controlled. This sort of patient will also prefabricate urine tests in order to mislead his doctor. This is obviously a stupid, immature type of approach that courts disaster. Without mutual understanding and trust it becomes that much more difficult for a diabetic to keep himself healthy and well.

Equally as important, any diabetic must have at least a basic understanding of the nature of diabetes. So often, patients display their ignorance by making statements such as: 'Have I still got sugar in my blood, doctor?', or 'There is sugar in my urine but I am sure there is none in my blood'. As explained in Chapter 1, the urine sugar is a simple reflection of the blood sugar and all of us have sugar in our blood. It is only a matter of degree whether we are diabetic or not. Therefore, statements such as those above reflect patient ignorance.

How can a diabetic begin to keep himself controlled and healthy if he doesn't understand the basic facts of what the urine tests really mean and what the blood sugar level really means? It is not good enough to feel well, since many diabetic complications occur without symptoms of poor diabetic control being present.

We have already discussed the major role played by inheritance in diabetes. Therefore all diabetics should urge their first degree relatives to be tested for diabetes every few years. This way, any unexpected and unsuspected diabetics can be diagnosed and their blood sugars controlled, possibly delaying the onset of long term complications.

Exercise is most important to anyone, diabetic or not. However, the diabetic on insulin will benefit even more from exercise than most people. Exercise will lower the blood sugar level by potentiating the action of insulin, so that if you are a diabetic on insulin, regular exercise will not only keep you physically fit and healthy, but will also aid in keeping your blood sugar down to normal levels. Remember, however, that excess exercise can produce fairly severe hypoglycaemic reactions and therefore you must always eat prior to and just after exercise. Cheese and biscuits or a sandwich are good supplements and are preferred to chocolate or candies, although glucose sweets should be on hand just in case the drop in blood sugar is more than anticipated and hypoglycaemia ensues. You will soon learn exactly how much extra food is necessary to cope with certain degrees of exercise. There are many professional sportsmen who are diabetics on insulin. To mention just one patient in particular – a 23-year-old man who is a Second Dan karate expert. He is superbly fit, working during the day, teaching karate in the evenings and participating in competitions. He has his dietary adjustment down to a fine art, knowing exactly how much to eat depending on whether he is training, teaching or competing in karate, so that both before and after the exercise he is always free of glycosuria, yet never goes hypoglycaemic. Not all diabetics can reach this degree of expertise, but the point is that exercise should not cause untoward problems in diabetic control if it is approached with intelligence. The maturity onset diabetic not on insulin needs exercise just as much as the insulin-requiring diabetic. Not only will the exercise help decrease the blood sugar, but it is an essential addition to a diet for weight loss. If you are over fifty, however, check with your doctor as to the amount of exercise you can safely do. The object is to make you fit, not to precipitate a heart attack!

The importance of urine testing cannot be overstressed. Many diabetics stop testing their urines because they find they are free of glycosuria all the time. It is all very well to be able to 'feel' when the sugar is high, but usually by the time symptoms of uncontrolled diabetes are recognized, the blood sugar is very high. It is nearly impossible to detect slight rises in blood sugar with moderate amounts of sugar in the urine. Therefore, if the urine is clear of sugar this is all the more reason to keep testing, since an increase in urinary sugar levels will be quickly detected before there is a major loss of diabetic control, and this can then be rectified early.

Recently there has been a move to teach certain diabetics to control their diabetes by testing their own blood sugar. This is done by a drop of blood from a finger prick, using commercially available glucose-measuring sticks (such as Dextrostix) and relatively inexpensive home machines. This certainly has its advantages in some situations, since, as previously discussed, sugar usually appears in the urine when the blood sugar is above 180 mg%. Since the normal blood sugar level is well below this (and never above 160 mg%) it is possible to have persistently slightly elevated blood sugar levels and yet never show sugar in the urine. This has been rather aptly described as trying to drive a car in a 50 miles per hour speed limit zone with a speedometer that only starts registering at 70 miles per hour. In most stable diabetics who remain free of sugar in the urine and who are seeing their doctors fairly regularly, the urine glucose test is nevertheless probably adequate. However, in certain instances, such as the pregnant diabetic, where very accurate diabetic control is essential (see Chapter 7) the idea of testing one's own blood sugar at home may prove particularly useful.


The diabetic balance

It must be evident by this stage that there are 3 major variable factors in the overall control of any insulin requiring diabetic. These are:

(1) Diet

(2) Insulin dose

(3) Individual variation – dependent upon the degree of activity, exercise, emotional state and mental outlook of any one person.

Obviously, it would be theoretically possible to attain perfect diabetic control if all three factors could be kept absolutely constant. Equally obviously, this is impossible, particularly with regard to the individual variations. Clearly, the amount of exercise and emotional stress varies not only day by day, but hour by hour. If, however, diet and insulin are kept constant, there is only one factor varying, so that an overall balance is still relatively easy to attain. On the other hand, if the diet is also inconsistent, there are two variables and only one constant (insulin dosage), so that overall balance becomes nearly impossible. Varying the insulin dose and the diet makes diabetic control completely impossible to achieve. Figure 9 demonstrates the great importance of correct diet and a consistent insulin dose.

Foot care

It is important to take great care of your feet. Because of involvement of the nerves to the feet a diabetic may not be able to feel discomfort or heat or pain in the feet as well as a non-diabetic. Furthermore, because of poor circulation to the extremities so commonly found in diabetics, small wounds to the feet often become infected and do not heal well. Therefore, a diabetic is more liable to develop ulcers, minor wounds and infections. Even when these develop, the diabetic will very often feel no pain and therefore remain unaware of the ulcer until it has extended considerably and gangrene has set in.

These complications can usually be prevented by care. It is most important to keep your feet clean and dry and to get

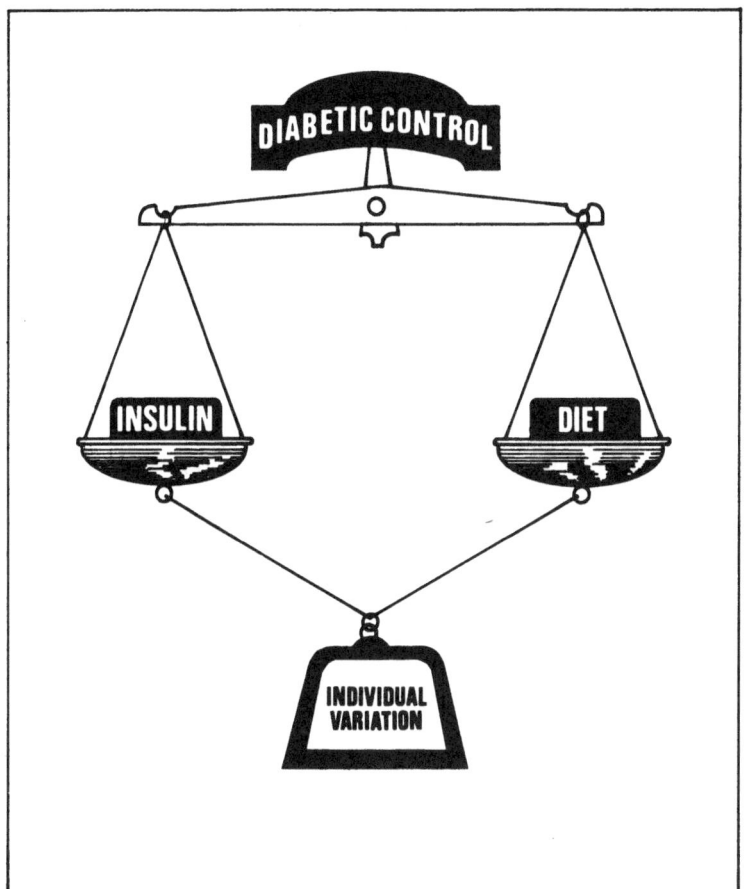

**Figure 9**

into the habit of inspecting your feet every evening both on the tops of the feet and under the soles to detect any cracks, cuts or ulcers. Shoes and socks must be comfortable and never tight, and blisters from badly fitting footwear must be avoided. Corns, callouses and bunions should not be cut or filed except by an expert and every diabetic should visit a chiropodist to attend to these problems. Toe nails should be cut straight across after being softened in warm water. If any difficulties are experienced in this, a chiropodist should be consulted. In any event, if you are known to have poor circulation or areas of numbness to your feet, it is probably a good idea to have your nails cut by a chiropodist in the first place. Any small injury, ulcer or sore on the foot or lower leg must be reported immediately to your doctor. In addition, any soggy white skin or discomfort between the toes should be reported. Athlete's foot should not be regarded lightly as this often becomes secondarily infected. Excessive heat must be avoided and in particular you must be very careful of hot water bottles or heating pads which could burn your feet during the night without you being aware of it (because of diminished sensation in the feet). If a hot water bottle must be used, it should be wrapped completely in thick flannel before use. Heating pads should be turned to a low heat if they are used. Never wear elastic or tight socks around the legs as this can diminish circulation even further.

Personal identification

All diabetics should carry a diabetic identification card or, preferably, wear a metal bracelet or pendant such as that obtainable from Medic-Alert. This is even more essential for the diabetic on insulin. This way, should anything happen such as a motor vehicle accident, or should you go unexpectedly into a diabetic coma and be unable to give a history, the medical attendant will immediately know you are diabetic and be able to institute correct treatment. This is a simple point but it can be life saving and should not be ignored. Many medicines interact with tablets taken for diabetes and many contain sugar so that it is important to take medicines only when prescribed by a physician.

Diabetic associations

Diabetes is a condition which is being researched extensively throughout the world and rapid advances are being made in the understanding and treatment of this disorder. It is therefore important to subscribe to the local diabetic association which will keep you informed of talks and lectures being held in the area and will post regular publications, so that you can keep in touch with recent developments in diabetes. This will also help you gain further insight and understanding into the condition. You must never think that you know all there is to know about diabetes. Often the patient who has been diabetic for 15 to 20 years is the most poorly controlled, having developed incorrect injection techniques and bad dietary habits, so that he inadvertently accepts poor diabetic control as a way of life. Familiarity breeds contempt and this must not be allowed to happen as it can prove fatal.

Finally, every diabetic should have a physical examination at least once a year and visit a dentist regularly. Often, particularly in diabetics on insulin, medical check-ups are warranted more regularly.

# Chapter Ten

## *Emotional factors and general considerations*

As any diabetic knows, diabetes forces one into a pattern of being constantly aware of one's illness so that the diabetes becomes completely enmeshed into day to day living. The implications of diabetes in the lives of patients are all.encompassing – from simple food preferences to major decisions regarding marriage, career, and holiday planning. Each diabetic will cope with his illness in a highly individual way. Usually, there are three basic well recognized patterns:

(1) *Rejection* – Unfortunately, many diabetic patients, reject their diabetes. ('If I pretend it doesn't exist, maybe it will go away.') This is a completely irrational approach and usually is present in patients who lack a complete understanding of the disorder, often because they don't want to know. As must already be evident, people who adopt this approach to their diabetes will sooner or later head for disaster. Unfortunately, these patients, being the very ones who most urgently need advice and treatment, are just the patients who shun doctors. This attitude is most often seen in teenage diabetics, probably as part of the 'adolescent revolt'. Fortunately, most of these patients eventually develop a more mature attitude and it is not uncommon for diabetics in their late teens or early twenties to present rather sheepishly to a doctor, asking to be disciplined and stabilized. If you have diabetes, the sooner you come to terms with it, accept it and adapt your lifestyle accordingly, the happier, healthier and more emotionally stable you will become.

(2) *Obsession* – A small proportion of diabetic patients take their diabetes so seriously that they read avidly any material on the subject (a good thing, if approached with the right mental attitude), test their urine eight times a day, count calories to the last one and measure carbohydrate, protein and fat intake to the final crumb. Clearly, this approach will lead these people into a completely regimented, unaltering and extremely dull lifestyle. While they may assure themselves of a longer healthier life, the anxiety engendered by this obsession makes both them and the people around them unhappy, and certainly reduces the quality of life. This sort of strict regimentation is really not necessary. One young diabetic man was so obsessive that he tested his urine every 2 hours, reacting completely irrationally at the first sign of sugar in the urine. The anxiety itself was sufficient to increase the blood sugar level so that his diabetes was extremely brittle. He then injected himself with extra insulin to counteract this, sometimes injecting himself 5 or more times a day. His diabetes ruled his life to the extent that he had no time or interest in any other activity, had no friends and had great difficulty in maintaining a job. After intensive psychiatric counselling he was instructed to test his urine once a day only. He kept this up for only one week before breaking down completely and reverting to his previous pattern. This unfortunate patient still remains as obsessive as ever and has reconciled himself to this, despite all attempts to wean him of this habit.

(3) *Intelligent acceptance* – This is by far the most healthy approach to the diabetic state. Certainly, if one has diabetes, one has to live with it, but with intelligent forethought and insight it soon becomes evident that apart from minor alterations in lifestyle there is nothing stopping any diabetic from living a normal, fulfilling and varied life.

Most diabetics, more usually those whose diabetes is diagnosed when young adults, go through all three of the above stages. Initially, at the time that the diabetes is diagnosed, there is a period of complete rejection. Sooner or later, however, the diabetic realizes that the disease will not just go away, and he becomes concerned about his health and passes into the obsessive phase. Soon after, however, with further understanding and insight into his diabetes, most diabetics pass into the third phase, that of acceptance, in which they remain. Problems in this regard only exist in diabetics who do not evolve beyond stages one or two.

While the stresses and strains of modern life impose emotional responses in all of us, it is important for the diabetic to realize the profound effect which emotion can have on diabetic control. This can be divided into direct and indirect effects on the blood sugar level.

## The direct effect of emotion on blood sugar

Frequently, the question is asked whether diabetes can be caused by a major emotional upset. Currently, there is very little room for the inclusion of emotional stress as a single or primary cause of active diabetes. A severe emotional shock could conceivably play a role in precipitating diabetes in someone who has been born with the predisposition to the disease, but in these people the diabetes would have occurred sooner or later anyway.

The majority of diabetics, particularly those on insulin, are well aware of the havoc which may be wrought on diabetic control by emotional upsets. The degree of loss of diabetic control varies from individual to individual, but all diabetics will be aware that major psychological stress will inevitably result in a transient loss of diabetic control. It is obviously impossible and even ridiculous to suggest that emotional upheavals be avoided – we would all avoid them if we could. Rather, accept the loss of diabetic control if the upset is short lived, and make the necessary adjustments in insulin dosage if it is likely to be a situation lasting longer than a few days. Emotional upsets cause the body to secrete an increased amount of anti-insulin hormones such as adrenalin and cortisone, which can be relatively easily countered by increasing the insulin dosage proportionately.

*Indirect effects of emotions on diabetes*

Inevitably, most diabetics will go through a phase where they become irritated and disenchanted with their diabetes and the constant care which they have to give themselves. At these times, there may be lapses in management and attention resulting in failure to test the urine or in dietary indiscretions. These spells may occur by chance but frequently there are a number of precipitating situations such as an unresolving life crisis, anxiety states, or depression. This most frequently occurs in the rebellious adolescent but can occur at any time of life. Self discipline becomes a major factor at these times, and if the diabetic has managed to incorporate his diabetic management into his lifestyle as a habit, these lapses can be avoided.

Marriage and the diabetic patient

Whatever one's feelings about marriage may be in these modern times, there is no doubt that marriage is an excellent institution for a diabetic patient. It provides the diabetic with a regular, more disciplined home life and increased protection, care, and psychological and physical support supplied by the spouse. When a diabetic marries, it is of course essential for the non-diabetic partner to understand as much about diabetes and management as does the diabetic. He or she must be prepared to cooperate in the management of the spouse's disease. The role of inheritance is described previously in Chapter 2 and it is abundantly clear that any children arising from the marriage are likely to be healthy and normal, and those who do develop diabetes usually will not do so until adulthood.

Sex and diabetes

Every diabetic can and should expect a full and normal sex life. Contraception is not a major problem in this regard, and the various types have already been discussed in Chapter 7. It has never been established that diabetes interferes with sexual enjoyment or performance in women diabetics. On the other hand, a well recognized complication of diabetes in men is impotence (the failure to attain or maintain an erection). This is due to involvement of the nerve to the penis in the diabetic neuritic process, and once it occurs it is usually permanent and does not respond to treatment. Very often, however, the fear of this complication results in psychological impotence in diabetic men, when there is no real physical problem. In fact, psychological impotence is probably far more prevalent than real physical impotence in diabetics. Unfortunately, it is extremely difficult to distinguish the one from the other. If true permanent impotence does occur, there are today several forms of surgery that can be performed to permit a functional 'artificial' erection to be achieved.

At times a temporary loss of libido or impotence may occur when the diabetes is uncontrolled. This is very different from the permanent impotence found with neuritis, and is probably due to the high sugar itself and the concurrent general poor health. With better diabetic control, sexual function will improve.

Rarely, another complication may occur. This is 'retrograde ejaculation'. There may be diabetic involvement of the nerve responsible for propelling the seminal fluid forwards along the penis, so that with orgasm the seminal fluid is ejaculated backwards into the bladder. One patient aptly described this as 'firing a blank'. This does not interfere with sexual enjoyment but can cause problems with fertility.

Despite these possibilities the vast majority of diabetic men enjoy a full, normal sex life. In most cases, no problems arise and none should be anticipated.

Diabetes is a unique disorder because, more than in any other illness, the patient has the responsibility of looking after himself. No matter how frequent the medical check-ups, no matter how excellent one's physician, diabetes will never be controlled and good health cannot be maintained without self care by the patient. The diabetic has to make daily decisions about his diet, exercise and insulin dosage. He must therefore understand the nature of his disease completely and learn what he can and cannot do without upsetting the control of his condition. Most people are able to integrate diabetes into their normal lives. As must be abundantly evident, some discipline has to become part of daily living, but the adversity of diabetes does not result in any major changes in lifestyle, nor need the diabetic deny himself the major enjoyments in life (other than gluttony and smoking). Accepting diabetes and its treatment will allow one to proceed in good health and in a happy and balanced state of mind.

# Appendix A

## Basic diets for those who want them

As I have stated elsewhere in this book, I do not believe in the adherence to rigid uncompromising diets. Nevertheless, the obese maturity onset diabetic does need to lose weight and maintain that weight loss as an integral part of treatment. Ideally, the diet should be individualized by a dietician, depending upon your individual age, body build and degree of overweight. Some patients are for one or other reason unable to obtain the services of a dietician and for these patients I present below a few recommended standardized 'average' diets which some might find useful.

The basic diets are outlined below. Lists of substitutes and food exchanges allowed are listed in Appendix C.

### 1200 CALORIE (5040 KILOJOULES) DIET FOR DIABETICS NOT ON INSULIN

This diet is recommended for the average overweight woman whose ideal body weight is in the region of 110 to 120 lbs (50 to 55 kilograms).

#### Foods that must be completely avoided

REFINED SUGAR in all its forms including candies, sweets, chocolates, glucose candies, peppermints and ice-cream.

CAKES, cookies, scones, pastries, biscuits, rusks, shortbread and rolls.

TINNED OR PRESERVED FRUITS, jellies, jams, marmalade, syrup, molasses and honey.

ALL PASTA including macaroni, spaghetti, vermicelli, noodles, thickened soups or gravies.

CHUTNEYS, sauces, pickles, hamburgers, sausages, polonies, pizzas.

DRIED PEAS, beans, lentils, barley, corn flour, tapioca, sago.

SWEETENED FIZZY DRINKS, sodas, beer, stout, wines, fruit squashes.

MILK DRINKS including Milo, Ovaltine, Horlicks, milk shakes etc.

MADE UP DISHES including fish cakes, rissoles, or any dishes with flour, breadcrumbs or sugar added.

FRIED FOODS of any kind including fried fish, frenchfries etc.

Daily ration of margarine = 15 gms (1 tablespoon).

Daily ration of skim milk = 250 ml (½ pint or 1 cup) –distributed in tea, coffee or cereal.

*The intake of eggs should be limited to a maximum of three (3) per week.*

| BREAKFAST: | This is a Most Important Meal and Must be Taken |
|---|---|
| Fruit | 1 portion, or substitute |
| Bread | 1 slice ¼ inch thick or substitute |
| Egg | 1, (boiled, poached or scrambled) or substitute |
| Margarine for bread | from daily ration |
| Tea or coffee | 1 cup – NO SUGAR |
| Milk for tea or coffee | from daily ration |

*LUNCH:*

| | |
|---|---|
| Meat | 90 gms (3 oz) cooked, or substitute |
| Large mixed salad | use vegetables from free group listed in Appendix C |
| Bread | 1 slice-¼ inch thick, or substitute |
| Margarine for bread | from daily ration |
| Fruit | 1½ portions, or substitute |
| Sweetmilk cheese | 30 gms (1 oz) (Block 2″ × 1″ × 1″) |

*DINNER:*

| | |
|---|---|
| Meat | 90 gms (3 oz) cooked, or substitute cooked any way except fried |
| 'Heavy' vegetable | 1 portion, or substitute |
| Free vegetable | 1 large serving from free vegetables |
| Fruit | 2 portions or substitute |

*BETWEEN MEALS:* i.e. mid-morning and mid-afternoon

Tea or coffee    1 cup – using milk from daily ration

*NO SUGAR AND NOTHING TO EAT*

If necessary, use saccharine or other artificial sweeteners.

*NOTES:*

Each meal is important.

Prepare the meal in different ways but do not change the quantities given.

If you keep strictly to this diet you will lose weight slowly. If you change the amounts, you will only put on weight, even if you eat less than is indicated.

## 1600 CALORIE (6720 KILOJOULES) DIET FOR DIABETICS NOT ON INSULIN

This diet is recommended for the average overweight man whose ideal body weight is in the region of 150 to 170 lbs (70 to 80 kilograms).

### Foods that must be completely avoided

REFINED SUGAR in all its forms including candies, sweets, chocolates, glucose candies, peppermints and ice-cream.

CAKES, cookies, scones, pastries, biscuits, rusks, shortbread and rolls.

TINNED OR PRESERVED FRUITS, jellies, jams, marmalade, syrup, molasses and honey.

ALL PASTA including macaroni, spaghetti, vermicelli, noodles, thickened soups or gravies.

CHUTNEYS, sauces, pickles, hamburgers, sausages, polonies, pizzas.

DRIED PEAS, beans, lentils, barley, corn flour, tapioca or sago.

SWEETENED FIZZY DRINKS, sodas, beer, stout, wines, fruit squashes.

MILK DRINKS including Milo, Ovaltine, Horlicks, milk-shakes etc.

MADE UP DISHES including fish cakes, rissoles, or any dishes with flour, breadcrumbs or sugar added

FRIED FOODS of any kind including fried fish, frenchfries etc.

Daily ration of margarine = 30 gms (2 tablespoons).

Daily ration of skim milk = 250 ml (½ pint) for distribution in tea, coffee or cereal.

*The intake of eggs should be limited to a maximum of three (3) per week.*

BREAKFAST: *This is a Most Important Meal and Must be Taken*

| | |
|---|---|
| Fruit | 1 portion or substitute |
| Cereal | 1 cup or substitute |
| Bread | 1 slice ¼ inch thick or substitute |
| Margarine | from daily ration |
| Egg | 1 or substitute |
| Tea or coffee | 1 cup – NO SUGAR |
| Milk for tea or coffee and cereal | from daily ration |

*LUNCH:*

| | |
|---|---|
| Meat | 90 gms (3 oz) cooked, or substitute |
| Large mixed salad | use vegetables from free group listed in Appendix C |
| Bread | 2 slices ¼ inch thick, or substitute |
| Margarine | from daily ration |
| Fruit | 1½ portions, or substitute |

*DINNER:*

| | |
|---|---|
| Meat | 90 gms (3 oz) cooked, or substitute |
| Potato | 90 gm (3 oz) cooked (1 medium), or substitute – to be served boiled or baked in jacket |
| Heavy vegetables | 1 serving |
| Free vegetables | 1 large serving |
| Fruit | 1 portion, or substitute |

NOTES:

Breakfast cereal means 1 cup of dry cornflakes or other patent flakes, except sugared ones *or* 1 cup cooked porridge.

MEAT, fish, potatoes and vegetables may be cooked in any way except fried in oil or fat.

White *or* brown bread may be eaten and may be toasted if desired. *Do not* buy diabetic bread as this is very expensive and is not necessary.

# Appendix B

## Diets for patients on insulin

Patients on insulin do not usually require a reducing diet, although they may be given one if they are overweight. The required calorie intake varies considerably for individuals depending upon age, sex, body build and degree of daily activity. Nevertheless, as a rough guide I have outlined below the sort of diet a young man or woman of average weight and average activity might require.

### DAILY DIET

Refined sugar in all its forms is totally prohibited, unless it is used to combat a hypoglycaemic reaction. Learn to manage without sugar completely, or use artificial sweeteners in its place. White or brown bread may be eaten and may be toasted if desired. Do not buy diabetic bread. This is very expensive and is not necessary.

*Do not eat more than three (3) eggs per week*

Daily ration of skim milk = 250 ml (½ pint – 1 cup) to be distributed in tea, coffee and cereal.

*BREAKFAST:*

| Food type | Men | Women |
|-----------|-----|-------|
| Fruit | 2 portions | 2 portions |

| | | |
|---|---|---|
| Bread or substitute | 2 portions | 1 portion |
| Egg or substitute | 1-2 portions | 1 portion |
| Margarine or substitute | 1-2 portions | 1 portion |

*MID-MORNING SNACK:* - See List - Appendix C

*LUNCH*:

| | | |
|---|---|---|
| Meat or substitute | 1-2 portions 90-180 gms | 1 portion 90 gms |
| Bread or substitute | 2 portions | 2 portions |
| Vegetables: free | Free | Free |
| restricted | 1 portion | 1 portion |
| Fruit | 1 portion | 1 portion |
| Margarine | 1-2 portions | 1 portion |

*MID-AFTERNOON SNACK* - See List - Appendix C

*DINNER:*

| | | |
|---|---|---|
| Meat or substitute | 1-2 portions 90-180 gms | 1 portion 90 gms |
| Bread or substitute | 2 portions | 2 portions |
| Vegetables: free | Free | Free |
| restricted | 1 portion | 1 portion |
| Fruit | 1 portion | 1 portion |
| Margarine or substitute | 1-2 portions | 1-2 portions |

*LATE-NIGHT SNACK* - See List - Appendix C

Alcohol intake to be limited as discussed in Chapter Three.

Artificially sweetened or 'diet' fizzy drinks are allowed as are sugar free fruit juices.

# Appendix C

## Food portions and substitutes

### One fruit portion =

| | | | |
|---|---|---|---|
| Apple - fresh | 1 medium | Orange | 1 small |
| Apple - dried | 4 rings | Orange Juice | ½ glass |
| Apricots - fresh | 2 average | Paw Paw | average slice |
| Apricots - dried | 6 halves | Peach - fresh | 1 medium |
| Banana | 1 medium | Peach - dried | 4 halves |
| Cherries | 10 large | Pear - fresh | 1 small |
| Coconut - fresh | 1" × 1" cube | Pear - dried | 4 halves |
| Figs - fresh | 2 large | Pineapple | ¾ inch slice |
| Fruit juice | ½ glass | Plums | 3 small |
| Gooseberries | ½ cup | Prunes - raw | 3 medium |
| Grapefruit | 1 large | Sponspek | 1 slice |
| Grapes | 12 | Strawberries | 1 cup |
| Guavas | 2 medium | Sweetmelon | 1 slice |
| Leechies | 3 medium | Watermelon | 1 large slice |
| Loquats | 4 medium | | |
| Manerines | 2 medium | | |
| Mangoes | 1 medium | | |
| Melon, cantalop | ½ small or cup cubed | | |
| Mixed fruit salad unsweetened | ½ cup | | |

### Free vegetables

Take as much of these as desired. They prevent you from feeling hungry and prove a very good source of vitamins and mineral salts.

Asparagus
Broccoli
Cabbage
Cauliflower
Celery
Cucumber
Eggplant
Gem squash
Green beans
Lettuce

Marrow
Mushrooms
Pepper
Radishes
Sauerkraut
Spinach
Spring onions
String beans
Tomatoes
Watercress

## Heavy vegetables

Artichokes = ½ cup

Beetroot = ½ average

Carrot = ½ average

Hubbard squash = ½ cup

Leeks = ½ cup

Mixed vegetables – peas,
carrots, corn and
green beans = ½ cup

Ocra = ½ cup

Parsnip = ⅓ average

Peas = 1 tablespoon

Pumpkin = ½ cup

Turnip = ½ average

Onion = 1 large or 2 small

## Free foods (can be used as desired)

Clear sour pickles
Lemon juice sweetened with artificial sweeteners
Rhubarb sweetened with artificial sweeteners

## Seasonings (may be used as desired)

Allspice

Bay leaves

Chopped parsley

Cinnamon

Mixed spices

Mustard

Nutmeg

Onion

| | |
|---|---|
| Garlic | Pepper |
| Lemon juice | Thyme & sage |
| Mint | Vinegar |

*SUBSTITUTES*

## Substitutes for meat

120 gm (4 oz) cooked fish
¾ cup salmon or tuna (canned and drained)
3 medium sardines (drained)
50 gm (approximately 5) small clams or shrimps
3 thin slices of salami
1 frankfurter or medium size sausage
average helping of chicken
2 eggs
60 gm (2 oz) sweetmilk cheese
2 tablespoons peanut butter

## Substitute for one egg

60 gm cooked fish
60 gm cooked liver
30 gm cheddar cheese
30 gm lean bacon (1 rasher)
½ of one meat portion or exchange

## Substitute for one slice bread

1½ portions fruit
4 creamcracker biscuits
1 medium potato
3 level tablespoons cooked rice
¾ cup patent cereal (e.g. cornflakes)
½ medium hamburger bun
½ cup cooked porridge
3 Graham crackers 2½ inches square

2 Ryecrisp breads (4" × 3")
½ cup thick soup (not for reducing diets)
½ cup ice-cream (not for reducing diets)
¼ cup cooked pasta
1 cob of corn
½ cup cooked kidney, lema or navy beans
1 cup popcorn (not for reducing diet)
30 gm (1 small packet) potato crisps (not for reducing diet)
2 rounds (8 cm) wholewheat crackers
¼ sheet matzos
3 tablespoons custard (made with skim milk)

## Substitute for one fruit portion

½ cup unsweetened patent cereal
½ cup cooked porridge
2 level tablespoons cooked rice
2 portions of cooked 'heavy' vegetables
⅔ of any of the exchanges of 1 slice bread

## Substitute for one cup milk

1 cup yoghurt
1 cup buttermilk

## Substitute for one teaspoon margarine

1 rasher bacon
3 medium olives
1 tablespoon whipped cream

*BETWEEN MEAL SNACKS FOR PATIENTS ON INSULIN*

Any one of the following may be taken

1 slice bread + peanut butter + ½ cup milk
1 portion fruit + cup milk

2 cream crackers + 1 cup milk
1½ slices bread + cheese *or* peanut butter
3 cream crackers + cheese *or* peanut butter
1 small piece sponge cake (no jelly or frosting) + ½ cup milk
1 small packet potato chips + cup milk
1 plain doughnut (small) + cup milk
¾ cup popcorn
¾ cup ice-cream

# Appendix D

## *Emergency diets*

The following are sample menus that may be used under emergency conditions. Using these samples, the patient should be able to make up other menus to suit his own likes and needs.

### Clear liquid diet

1½ quarts of 10% fruit juice such as orange or pineapple juice or ginger ale taken at hourly intervals over a 24 hour period. This provides 150 grams of carbohydrates

### Liquid diet (150 grams carbohydrate)

| Time | Food | Amount |
|---|---|---|
| 8:00 a.m. | orange juice | 1 cup |
| 10:00 a.m. | eggnog<br>1 cup milk<br>1 egg<br>1 teaspoon sugar<br>½ drop vanilla | one |
| 12:00 noon | beef broth | ½ cup |
| | milk | 1 cup |
| 2:00 p.m. | ginger ale | 1 bottle 6 oz |
| 4:00 p.m. | pineapple juice | 1 cup |

| 6:00 p.m. | chicken broth | ½ cup |
|-----------|---------------|-------|
| | milk | 1 cup |
| 8.00 p.m. | grape juice | ¾ cup |
| 10:00 p.m. | cocoa made with milk<br>1 teaspoon sugar | 1 cup |

Times for taking liquids may vary as long as this much food is consumed in 24 hours.

## Soft (bland) diet

| Time | Food | Amount |
|------|------|--------|
| 8:00 a.m. | unsweetened fruit juice | ½ cup |
| | cooked cereal | ½ cup |
| | milk | ½ cup |
| 10:30 a.m. | egg (scrambled or soft boiled) | one |
| | bread, toasted | 1 slice |
| | margarine | 1 pat |
| | milk | ½ cup |
| 12:00 noon | thick soup | ½ cup |
| | crackers | two |
| | cottage cheese | ½ cup |
| | fruit | one portion |
| | bread | 1 slice |
| 3:00 p.m. | custard | ½ cup |
| | milk | ½ cup |
| 5:30 p.m. | broiled burger patty | one |
| | potato (baked or boiled) | one medium |
| | soft cooked carrots | ⅓ cup |
| | milk | ½ cup |
| | butter or margarine | |
| 8:00 p.m. | applesauce or fruit juice (unsweetened) | ½ cup |
| 10:00 p.m. | cocoa or ½ cup ice-cream | |

*NOTE:*

If you are on insulin, take your usual dose, or more if the urine contains more sugar than usual. Although your food intake is reduced, the acute illness may require an increase in insulin dosage and some patients may be instructed by their doctor to take additional regular insulin in emergencies. Vomiting is dangerous in diabetics and if this persists or is associated with shortness of breath it needs urgent medical attention.

# Index